CHRIS SHELTON'S
EASY GUIDE TO FIX
NECK
AND
BACK
PAIN

CHRIS SHELTON'S
EASY GUIDE TO FIX
NECK
AND
BACK
PAIN

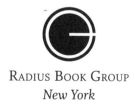

RADIUS BOOK GROUP
New York

Radius Book Group
A division of Diversion Publishing Corp.
www.radiusbookgroup.com

Radius Book Group and colophon
are registered trademarks of Diversion Publishing Corp.
For more information, email info@radiusbookgroup.com

First Radius Book Group Edition: September 2024
Hardcover ISBN: 978-1-63576-922-7
Trade Paperback ISBN: 978-1-63576-940-1
e-ISBN: 978-1-63576-929-6

Design by Neuwirth & Associates, Inc.
Illustrations: Chris Shelton
Model: Nare Israelyan
Line editor and copyeditor: Nichole Gates
Photographers: Heidi Cox and Chris Schmauch
Graphic designer: Josh Orenstein
Headshot: Gregory Zabilski
For more information, email news@sheltonqigong.com

Printed in the United States of America
1   3   5   7   9   10   8   6   4   2

▪ ▪ ▪

EXTRA RESOURCES

To give you the best experience with this book, my team and I have created an online resource that includes my Five Element Questionnaire as well as detailed descriptions of the different personality types.

You will find a copy of these and the rest of your resources by scanning the QR code below or by visiting this website:

www.chrissheltonseasyguide.com

■ ■ ■

DEDICATION

When you take things for granted, like being able to go to the bathroom and wipe your bottom or put on your tennis shoes and then, sadly, those abilities are taken away, you see the value of your spine in daily life.

Having suffered debilitating back pain more than once and experienced not being able to do these things or even walk, I dedicate this book not to one particular person but to the millions of people who have suffered or are still suffering from chronic neck and lower back issues.

I'm thankful for the guidance and knowledge given to me by the many teachers I mention in the acknowledgments section toward the end of this book.

I'm also thankful for the people in my life who have helped me compile this ancient wisdom in combination with modern medicine to show others that there is an answer and a way out of pain.

For anyone who has suffered or is only beginning to experience chronic neck and back issues, I hope the material offered here will give you a deeper insight into how your spine functions in coordination with your emotions, diet, lifestyle habits, and environment.

I hope you will use these tools and recommendations to heal yourself— and if you know someone who is suffering, please share this information.

I always say that I don't enjoy being sick or in pain, and I also don't like to see other people suffering or in pain.

I hope you are inspired by my journey. Know that I've been in your position and that there is a way to heal yourself and live a pain-free life.

May you live the glorious life that you were meant to. Be well and be blessed.

—Chris Shelton

CONTENTS

. . .

FOREWORD

by Billy Blanks

Founder of Tae Bo Fitness
9th degree black belt in Tae Kwon Do
4th degree black belt in Hung Gar Choy Gar Fu Gar

Some people have a preconception about Chinese medicine. There will always be those who are skeptical about new or different ways of thinking, but I want to assure you that you don't have to be Asian to adopt this mindset.

Chris is a healer who works from the inside out. Western thinking tends to focus only on physical manifestations, but it's so refreshing to find someone who starts by mending the true spirit first.

I found Chris through Eric the Trainer. We connected, and he asked how he could help. Chris talked to me about Qi, which I knew about from studying Chinese Hung Gar Choy Gar Fu Gar from Master Ting Fong Wong (Golden Dragon, Buffalo, New York) and from studying Tae Kwon Do from Grand Master Park Jong-Soo.

The first time Chris put his hands on me I was like, "Oh my God!" I didn't know what was blocked, but I could feel it coming out. When I got up, I could walk, jump, kick, and do splits after having had a bad hip since I was 18 years old.

Before that I would force myself to move through the pain and I just kept making everything worse. Then I got the chance to go to Chris. It was amazing. I started telling people about him, and I haven't looked back. I ended up playing in an NFL Super Bowl celebrity game. I would never have been able to do that if it weren't for Chris's help.

I've noticed that when I'm in Chris's house or even just near him, I can feel the presence of God. God works through him. Chris is not scared to do God's work. He doesn't hide His presence. That's what happens when you're around people who have a calling. When God works through a healer, you can feel it when you walk into a room. You can feel the Oneness.

I don't think things happen by accident. I know that I was meant to meet Chris.

As you read this book, remember that words control your destiny. Underline and memorize his words so that when trouble comes, instead of listening to your own thoughts or worries, you'll speak and remember his healing words. Have faith and trust. The power of faith that comes through Chris heals people; a higher purpose works through him. You need to know the spirit of the healer and understand his mind and his authority over sickness and disease. That's the purpose of this book.

Have faith and believe that when you walk in to see Chris or read his words, he *can* facilitate healing in you and also teach you how to heal yourself.

■ ■ ■

INTRODUCTION

Back pain is no joke.

If you've ever had a serious back injury, you've realized very quickly just how much our backs do for us.

Simple things you take for granted, like tying your shoes, standing up straight, being able to take a deep breath, and even wiping your bottom while going to the bathroom, are major tasks when you have severe lower back pain. And you're not alone.

According to WebMD, Americans spend approximately $86 billion each year trying to fix back issues. In fact, 80 percent of all adults experience low back pain at some point in their lives. It's the leading contributor to missed days of work and job-related disabilities. If you're currently experiencing back pain or if you've suffered from it in the past, you know how agonizing it is!

Back pain is a costly and debilitating disease that does not discriminate between athletes and couch potatoes, young and old, male and female. According to Western medicine, the causes of back pain include age, prolonged sitting, certain occupations—especially those involving heavy lifting or twisting and bending—being overweight, and even diabetes (that's because diabetes affects the way the body uses blood sugar, which in turn can damage the nerves that exit the spinal canal, creating pain, numbness, tingling, and atrophy).

Even though I say back pain doesn't discriminate, I've noticed in my 20 years of clinical experience that the elderly and women are more prone to back-related issues. There are many studies that support my observations. Regardless, if you're here and looking for a solution, you're in the right place.

In the '70s and '80s when I was growing up, it seemed as if the only people who complained of back pain or sciatica were those who were sedentary or obese. Today I have some clients whose primary care doctors tell them that they must lose weight and strengthen their core muscles in order to get rid of their back pain. While it's true that they should lose some weight and it does help to strengthen the core, neither of those issues is really the culprit.

I came to this understanding after working with thousands of clients. In this book, I'm going to teach you what I've learned about the two main causes of back pain, how to get immediate relief on your own, and the key lifestyle adjustments you can make that will help prevent your back pain from sneaking up again in the future.

HOW TO GET THE MOST FROM THIS BOOK

This is your handbook for understanding the root causes of neck, mid-, and low back pain, and a guide to fixing these issues yourself. As you will see, there's a lot of information—the root causes of disease and how we get sick, Qigong basics, how emotions affect our health, yin-yang principles, and the Five Elements theory.

I've also included sections on the functions of the internal organs as well as what dysfunctions look like when the organs are out of balance. The real meat of this book is found in the tools and techniques that will empower you to heal your neck and back yourself.

So if you're in chronic pain and need help right away, jump to part 2 of the book and learn how to fix things like cervical arthritis, lumbar stenosis, drop-leg syndrome, frozen shoulder, and side stitch.

Then I suggest you go back and read chapters 1 and 2, which talk about the root causes of disease, diet and nutrition, your DNA, and emotional health. These are the culprits in the majority of back conditions that I see in my clinical practice.

From there, I recommend taking the Five Element Questionnaire to find out your primary typology and what you're deficient in, because this will give you a heads-up as to what type of back pain you may be more prone to.

I recommend going to www.chrissheltonseasyguide.com and downloading the multiple charts that describe your element typology, what it looks like when you're out of balance, and what you can do to restore balance.

Then order my first book, *Chris Shelton's Easy Guide to Emotional Well-Being with Qigong*, 3rd ed., and go to sheltonqigong.com and provide your email address to receive other tools that will empower you to live your ultimate life.

My first book will give you further detailed instructions on the Qigong prac-tices that I recommend throughout this book and on my YouTube channel.

A NOTE ON CAPITALIZATION

You'll see throughout this book that when I'm talking about the internal organs, sometimes they will be capitalized and sometimes not.

When talking about the organ itself and its functions according to West-ern medicine, I don't capitalize the word.

When discussing energetic attributes and functions of the internal organs according to Chinese medicine—like the Liver, for example, and how it's most active between 1:00 and 3:00 a.m. or that it houses the spiritual com-ponent of the Ethereal Soul—then I capitalize the word.

PART ONE

CHINESE MEDICINE AND ACHIEVING VIBRANT HEALTH

QIGONG BASICS

What is Qigong (chee-gung)?

Qigong is a 5,000-year-old Chinese exercise system that teaches one how to harness the life force energy that permeates all things. It allows you to improve and balance your physical, mental/emotional, and spiritual health and prolong the quality of your life. When the system is properly in balance and flow, we can begin to alleviate chronic ailments, including chronic neck and back pain.

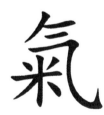

Qi refers to the life force energy that exists in all things, material and nonmaterial. Everything you see and don't see is an expression of this energy. Qi is an extension of matter and includes what appears to be nonexistent, the apparent and the non-apparent. It is also referred to as the "unmanifest." The center of space and time itself is an expression of Qi.

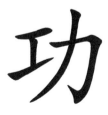

Gong is the art and practice of tapping into this life force energy; it is a learned skill. It involves understanding the connection between your internal organs and your emotions as well as becoming aware of your outside environment and how it affects you on the inside and vice versa. Our internal organs, our emotions, and the way we respond to our environment play a major role when the body goes out of balance. We must consider the role these factors play in order to properly understand and remedy physical pain in the body.

The concept of Qi is at the heart of classical Chinese medicine theory, and Qigong-type exercises are as old as the medicine itself. The fact that Chinese medicine has been around for more than 5,000 years is, in itself, evidence that it works. History has shown that anything fake or false inevitably reveals its flaws over time and is discarded.

According to the sages of ancient times, Qi is the energy that creates, infuses, and sustains all life. Qi is present and expressed through all things, including inanimate objects like rocks, living things like plants and animals, and the subtle states of immaterial things like air, light, sound, and thought.

The ancient Chinese devised a universal system to describe the various forms of energy, not only in the human body and the weather but also in space (through landscape and geography) and over time (in history and astrology). By understanding that everything in the cosmos is an expression of Qi, from the material to the insubstantial, we can glimpse the ultimate truth of the universe so we may come into a deep understanding and appreciation of the natural world, including our true nature.

You can experience Qi for yourself by simply taking one conscious breath—because breath is your Qi. Everything around you is an expression of Qi, whether you can see it or not, because Qi includes the tangible and the intangible. From the smallest atom to the vast universe, it is all an expression of Qi in different states of aggregation.

This is an important thing to consider when we look at something like neck and back pain. If all "form" is an expression of Qi, then Qi is also the basis of our internal physical structures. Qigong and Chinese medicine incorporate this knowledge into their ancient healing modalities in order to more effectively return harmony to our bodies.

There is only one Qi, but based on its function, different names are assigned to it, such as life force, energy, or vitality. If Qi is strong and coherent, life flourishes. If Qi becomes stagnant, deficient, or scattered, this opens the door for disease and, ultimately death. Qigong is a means of working with, cultivating, and developing our personal energy systems, and with a strong energetic foundation, our bodies can maintain balance and alignment, allowing us to remedy and heal chronic pain and inflammation.

THE THREE SCHOOLS
OF QIGONG

There are three schools of Qigong: medical, martial arts, and spiritual. Qigong exercises and meditations are also referred to as Qigong self-regulation practices. These techniques are the foundation on which you will be able to work on yourself medicinally on all three levels—physically, emotionally, and spiritually. All three schools impact the total health of the body.

Even for something one might consider purely physical, like chronic neck and back pain, targeted movement of the body and changes on a spiritual level will impact overall recovery as much as the medical aspects of Qigong. The Qigong practices I share in this book and on our YouTube channel are meant to empower you to improve your health, heal and prevent disease, and prolong your life.

- **Curative Qigong**® (sometimes referred to as Medical Qigong) is the foundation of acupuncture. It applies increased sensitivity and awareness to the body, along with the theories of classical Chinese medicine, to prevent and reverse the disease process. Practitioners look at organ function and pathology, channel function and pathology, our genetics, how seasons and foods affect us, how we respond to emotions, how well we sleep, and more. They take everything into account to discover the root cause of the disharmony.

- **The Martial Arts School** of Qigong is any form of internal martial arts, such as Tai Chi (or Taiji), Taijiquan, *xing yi*, *baguazhang*, and others. It is based on internally cultivated power rather than brute force and teaches you how to move in alignment with the cosmos.

- **The Spiritual School** is not an ism or a formal religion. Rather, it's the understanding that you can refine, cultivate, and preserve your life force energy to transform yourself spiritually and dissolve the false self, or the ego. With dedicated practice, you can develop the potential to quiet the mind, reach enlightenment, and experience immortality.

In other words, as you refine your life essence from the gross physical states to the more refined subtle states, you will become closer to God, which will allow you to connect with the all-knowingness of the universe.

HOW QIGONG WORKS

To better understand this book's recommendations for addressing your chronic neck and back pain, it will help to have a little background on how this ancient practice works.

According to Chinese medicine, Qi flows in specific pathways in the body called *meridians*. Each meridian is associated with a particular organ. The meridians can be compared to rivers and the internal organs to lakes that are supplied and drained by these rivers. So as in nature, when an insufficient amount of water flows from a river, the lake it feeds will dry up, adversely affecting the surrounding environment and all related ecosystems. On the other hand, if too much water comes down the river, the lake will overflow, affecting the same environment and related ecosystems, but to their detriment. Using this metaphor, we can say that the purpose of Qigong is to balance and harmonize the rivers and lakes of the body so they function at peak capacity, allowing the entire ecosystem of the body, including the back and neck, to maintain proper movement and function.

■

Qigong is a method for maintaining your
vital life force. It is not based on belief—that is,
you don't have to believe in it for it to work.

■

Health is an expression of the smooth flow of life-giving Qi throughout the body. Disease manifests when the flow of Qi is blocked or stagnant or when there is too much or too little present in the body. The physical and mental exercises provided in this book can clear blockages, dissolve stagnation, reduce excesses, and supplement deficiencies to bring the balance we need to achieve greater health.

I often use the terms *excess* and *deficient* throughout this text because these are part of Chinese medical theory. They describe conditions in which there is too much of something or too little—that is, when an organ is hyperactive or is becoming weak or hypoactive. To add to the complexity, we can sometimes see both excessive and deficient patterns in the same organ system. Both excess and deficiency as well as the combination of the two create imbalances that lead to chronic conditions like neck and back pain. However, as each person is different, so is their body and its unique pathway to disease.

In these chapters, you will learn how to interpret the signs and signals your body sends you and how to correct and improve the flow of Qi. That is the practice and purpose of Qigong. It can benefit you and those you know personally as well as your clients or patients if you are a health care practitioner.

THE ROOTS OF DISEASE

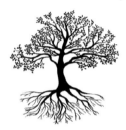

According to Chinese medicine, chronic neck and back pain have the same roots in basic dysfunction as all other disease in the body. When we look at the system as a whole, we see that the major causes of all disease, including physical ailments, are negative emotions, an unhealthy diet, and improper lifestyle habits.

Diet and emotions influence the body differently, but they ultimately interact. Diet supplies the physical substances from which the body continually recreates itself. Emotions determine the quality of the subtle energies of the body, which influence organ function. Based on observations made by physicians over thousands of years, we know that certain internal organs store unique negative emotions.

When these emotions are bottled up or expressed inappropriately, the proper function of their related organs is disrupted, causing chronic pain, disease, and sometimes fatal health problems. Certain organs store various kinds of energy and are damaged by excesses or deficiencies. This has whole-body consequences that can impact any part of the body related to these specific organs. A main principle of Chinese medicine and Qigong is that organ system dysfunction plays a critical role in all physical and emotional imbalances, including chronic neck and back pain.

I'm not saying that certain emotions are bad. That's not what I mean when I say "negative emotions." Rather, emotions are like a barometer. For example, anger is a good emotion if it inspires you to do something creative, fight for the underdog, get yourself out of a bad situation, or create positive change in the world. The same emotion becomes a negative force when the consequences are destructive to oneself or others.

People know when they are sick; they also know how they feel when they are well. This is an awareness of Qi. Practicing Qigong focuses on rediscovering this awareness. If we work to develop a greater capacity to perceive and address subtle signs of imbalance in the body, gross signals like chronic pain and discomfort will not arise.

Once we know that everything is connected, it might seem as if there are many moving parts to chronic neck and back pain. Which part of the body is sick? What is wrong with the Qi? Is it stuck? Is there too much or too little? Through practicing the meditations and gentle exercises of Qigong, we can answer these questions—and learn how to remedy the situation.

THE ROOTS OF EMOTIONAL HEALTH

Because we know internal organs are interrelated, we also know that dysfunctions in one organ can eventually lead to dysfunctions in another. Thus, in clinical practice, a practitioner can work backward from the disease that is manifesting to emotional or environmental toxins and find the true root of a condition. When we look at neck and back pain, we seek to discover the root of the pain, its beginnings, whereas the branch can be seen as the "fruit" of the disease, or the imbalance itself.

This is as true for neck and back pain as it is for any other symptom. Discovering the emotional and environmental toxins at the root of your body's imbalance will pinpoint the trigger for your physical pain.

Seen as a whole system, Chinese medicine includes the effects that thoughts and perceptions have on a person's physical well-being. For example, a main aspect of emotional health and overall physical wellness is one's attitude toward aging and beauty.

Aging is inevitable; we all must face a decline in our physical faculties. So often nowadays, we see people focusing on external beauty, having surgery or liposuction and using techniques like Botox in an attempt to preserve the fountain of youth. Sometimes even physical injuries can be traced back to excessive or improper attitudes and routines that were formed based on a desire to avoid the natural signs of aging.

Chinese medicine in general and Qigong in particular address this issue from two standpoints. First, the attitude: Why is a person so concerned about appearance? Is it because of fear? Envy? Ego? Exploring these questions can be important. When your organs are in harmony, you will feel so good—enjoying your life, your family, and your passions—that you will not have time for such states.

Second Qigong asks you to reassess what beauty means and to look within. When we look at a person's face, it tells us deep, hidden secrets about the personality, including how they think, what emotional traumas they have been through (and are still holding on to), and what potential diseases might be lurking. It is by working on these deep levels that true beauty can be revealed. In fact, if you want to look younger longer, practicing Qigong can actually help slow the aging process by freeing you from trauma stored within the body.

Using the wisdom of Qigong and Chinese medicine, we can achieve "ageless" beauty. When you are sleeping well and your organs (including your skin) are functioning correctly and not storing negative emotions or toxic digestive waste, you will radiate health and beauty—at any age. Without drastic measures, this beauty will translate to your entire body, down to the muscles, tendons, and ligaments. It will seem as though the whole body can maintain a greater level of suppleness and resilience, prolonging health and vitality throughout your life span.

Simple practices, profound results.

THE BENEFITS OF QIGONG

The meditations and exercises described in this book will certainly give your Qi a workout, but you will finish feeling revitalized and refreshed rather than worked out or exhausted. Each day of practice should bring greater and more significant benefits to help resolve the various neck and back issues that present themselves, gradually refining your health and vitality—your fundamental nature—and relieving your pain.

To our Western minds, it seems incredible that these simple movements and meditations can have such profound effects. No surgery? No drugs? But it's true. All you need is 15 minutes a day and, in a couple of weeks, you will notice this healing for yourself.

One of the greatest benefits of Qigong is that you will gradually become your own superior doctor, or practitioner. These practices will put you in touch with your body in subtle ways. You will develop a sensitivity to both the emotional and the physical conditions in your body. The whole idea is that eventually you will be able to detect disease before it sets in. Once you are in realignment and free from neck and back pain, you will recognize the first signs of imbalance, thus avoiding reinjury. Qigong teaches you how to listen to your internal wisdom and address dysfunction in its early stages so that the progression of chronic pain stops in its tracks.

With regular practice of the meditations and exercises described in this book, you will possess the tools to fix or prevent neck and back pain as well as other symptoms of disease—and the best part is, you'll know how to fix it yourself.

ARE YOU READY TO START HEALING YOUR BACK AND NECK PAIN?

Like I said,

Qigong is a simple practice with profound results.

I love that Qigong is such an all-encompassing practice. What's really groovy about it is that anybody can do it, even people who are feeling weak, are experiencing health issues, or are in a wheelchair. And it can be done from a seated or even a lying-down position.

You don't need a mat and you don't need expensive equipment. You don't have to wear fancy silk pajamas or a cloak. Wear anything that's comfortable. Do it indoors. Do it outdoors. Do it anytime.

If you have a hard time accepting the concept of Qi or the theories about how it works, then—like I did in the beginning—ignore it all! Just stick to the exercises.

Based on the successful experiences of countless generations of people who have used and passed down these exercises, give them a try. Observe carefully. Your body has its own wisdom as to how and when it heals. You may be surprised by what happens, and it may not happen as you expect it to. Simply practice consistently. Over time, you will experience greater vitality, health, and emotional well-being.

The whole idea of Qigong is to empower you to deal with stress and emotional trauma from the past and the present to rectify those emotional imbalances in the body that lead to disease. It's all about prevention and maintenance. Even when you do have something going on, these simple Qigong remedies can help pull you out of it. As your own superior doctor, you'll become so aware of your body, your connection to your environment, and the people around you that you will start to sense when something is out of balance or disease is setting in. In particular, if one of your internal organs gets out of balance, you will actually be able to notice it and rectify it before it leads to pain and inflammation.

Once you can feel what's going on anywhere inside your body, guess what? Your body will begin to talk to you. It will communicate when something's going wrong. And that's when you will use these practices, such as the five-organ cleansing exercise, white pearl meditation, microcosmic orbit meditation, and brushing the acupuncture meridians. These exercises will help bring balance to the underlying causes of chronic conditions like neck and back pain while preventing further issues from arising.

These tools and techniques are designed to help you achieve overall health and balance in your life. You will notice pain and inflammation subsiding, and on a deeper level, as you let go of your emotional baggage, you will also be letting go of the "coarse vibration" that most people walk around with. Our false selves or ego-selves tend to govern us—most of us, anyway. As you practice, those masks will start to fall away and you'll grow spiritually.

Because all is Qi, when you take steps to align and heal your neck and back pain, you are simultaneously taking positive steps toward your own spiritual development. It doesn't matter what religion you study or what spiritual tradition you practice. As you let go of this coarse vibration, your own authentic vibration increases and becomes more refined, or subtle. Your communication with God increases and your oneness with the universe grows, along with your own inner knowingness. Qigong does not differentiate between body, mind, and spirit. All three are in play when imbalance sets in, and all three achieve greater harmony when balance is restored.

Sometimes physical pains are associated with particular states of mind or even specific relationships in your life. As you increase your own authentic vibration, you may notice that people on a lower vibration (friends, family members, etc.) start to fall away. In the process, they may try to engage you negatively in an effort to hold on to you. However, as those people fall away, you'll continue to draw in others with a vibration similar to yours who will continue to uplift your spirit. This is a positive step in the healing process. As your body achieves greater wellness, healthier people and relationships will be drawn to you, while more negative ones will lose their hold.

One of my favorite quotes by Jim Rohn has to do with character building and success principles. He says, "In order to be beautiful, surround yourself with beautiful people. In order to be successful, surround yourself with people who are successful." (Note: he's not just referring to external beauty.) It follows that when we want to achieve greater health, surrounding ourselves with healthy people and relationships will support the work we are doing.

The journey of a thousand miles begins with a single step. Thanks for joining me on your own journey to healing your neck and back pain.

Let's get started!

▪ 2 ▪

UNDERSTANDING YIN AND YANG

AUTHOR'S NOTE

The goal of this chapter is to bring a greater understanding of the fundamental philosophy and theory behind Chinese medicine and Qigong to help close the gap between East and West so you can maximize the information in this book. Because yin and yang theory is so universal, I've chosen to include in this section only the principles that I feel are most important for the novice reader searching for a pain-free and balanced life. At the same time, I hope this section subtly awakens and reminds the more experienced practitioner of the importance of yin and yang in healing pain and disease.

This chapter will give you a glimpse into the simple beauty of the universe, including why opposites attract and why masculine and feminine energies form the perfect union. There are some tangible scientific examples to aid in your understanding; however, I am in no way trying to state that these scientific models and yin and yang philosophy are the same. They are two different, separate perspectives and thought processes—though yin and yang can be used to describe even our DNA and RNA.

Please be patient when reading this section. Its sole purpose is to show you how this ancient philosophy can be applied to your life. It's meant for people like you and me who are interested in personal growth and development—and when it comes to this book, how to resolve back pain. You may have heard of yin and yang but never before had a way to begin to grasp its deep and universal meaning or its role in all of life, including our physical health and well-being.

Although it gets technical at times, you will discover a few of the processes and patterns of the universe that will help you learn more about and expand into the best version of yourself. If you're reading this, your journey has already begun. Enjoy!

■ ■ ■

I grew up in San Jose, California. When I was a child, my family would take occasional trips to Santa Cruz, a California beach city. I remember seeing this symbol on some of the surfboards:

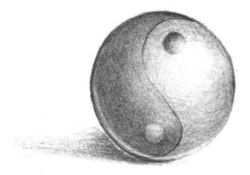

I was particularly drawn in by this image, which seemed to be universal. I realized at that time that emptiness and space are all *one*. It was deep thinking for an eight-year-old!

Then, when I was 19, I was introduced to the ancient art of Qigong and Tai Chi, which eventually changed the course of my life. One of the reasons Qigong is so powerful is that it's a practice that aims to balance not only the yin and yang of your body and environment but your entire life. This balance is key when you are looking to restore total health and alignment to the body, both in healing disease and preventing further disruption.

Clients with chronic pain frequently ask, "How can I experience joy when there is so much suffering in this life?" My answer is that if you can understand and practice natural energy flow, you will be able to access joy and harmony at any time, even in your darkest moments.

Yin and yang is an energy language that helps us understand this natural flow. The concept of yin and yang has been at the forefront of Chinese philosophy for centuries. For Western minds to understand this ancient theory, we must grasp the following basic concepts:

- NO-thing is what it seems.

- Every phenomenon in the multi-universe is an expression of Qi in grosser or finer vibrational frequencies.

- The paradox and duality of life can be described as yin and yang. Every event in the multi-universe is an interchanging, cyclical movement of these opposing and interconnected forces. It is the motivating force for change, transformation, and restoration.

■ ■ ■

If you stand still for a few moments with your eyes closed, you'll feel the pull of your inner yin and yang. One half of your body will lean or sway a little bit; this is a basic example of their presence. With this we realize that all things are, at all times, in a certain stage of flux and movement and that nothing is in a static state of 50-50.

THE NATURE OF YIN AND YANG

Yin and yang, though representing two apparent opposites, simultaneously exist within one another. They are interdependent. One cannot exist without the other. An example of this is the sun's rays, which can be viewed as pure yang energy. Without an opposite (yin) object, such as water, for the sun to bounce off, one would not be able to tell if the sun had rays or not.

Everything in the universe is in a constant state of change and development of consciousness. Even when the "apparent" is showing, the "non-apparent" is beginning to manifest. For example, in the coldest winter, when trees are covered with snow and the leaves have fallen off, it appears as though there is no life left in them (which would be considered yin). Yet if you look closely, you'll see the beginning of new life starting to sprout. Wiping the snow off the branches will reveal the next season's buds already starting to swell (a yang quality).

There is no aspect of life to which yin and yang do not apply. These two apparent opposites describe the interrelationship of everything known to humankind.

The qualities of yin and yang are relative, not absolute. What may be considered yang in one sense can sometimes be viewed as yin in another. For example, autumn is yang compared to the dead of winter but is considered yin when compared to midsummer.

YIN AND YANG BALANCE

Within nature, as within our bodies, yin and yang always seek to reach a natural state of equilibrium, and when one is thrown out of balance, the other is affected. For example, when yin is in excess, yang will, in turn, decrease. In the body, imbalances can become so severe that the body looks for its own solution to bring things into balance. This is where many of our symptoms of pain and disease arise. See table below.

Yang	Yin
Fire	Water
Hot	Cold
Restless	Quiet
Dry	Wet
Hard	Soft
Excitement	Inhibition
Rapid	Slow
Change	Storage
Day	Night
Summer	Winter
Up	Down
Positive	Negative
Masculine	Feminine
Qi	Blood

As an example, imagine that your yin is severely depleted. Your body will respond by forcing a situation that will bring balance. Exhaustion takes over and you begin to need more sleep or have a health crisis that compels you to slow down and rest. Although these physical symptoms are experienced as a negative, they are the body's attempt to restore stability.

According to the principle of constant change, nothing ever remains static at 50 percent yin and 50 percent yang. As yang declines, yin grows and vice versa. The result is a cycle of relative peaks and valleys in time, space, and density. Everything in the universe follows this pattern.

Here is an example: water in lakes and oceans is substantial matter. It heats up during the day and some is transformed into vapor, which is insubstantial. In the evening, the air cools and the vapor condenses back into water. Water and vapor are in a constant state of interplay and change as are yin and yang.

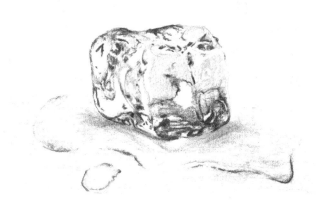

Life is never perfectly balanced or even like a straight line (Birth——Death). Instead, our lives are made up of peaks and valleys. See figures below.

Life of balance and consistency

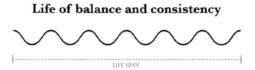

LIFE SPAN

Some people's lives are a series of extreme peaks, inevitably followed by steep declines. Extreme ups and downs will shorten your life span, so it is important to strive for balance.

Life of extremes

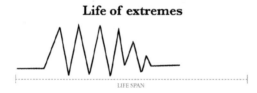

LIFE SPAN

Yin and yang continually transform into one another. For example, summer changes into winter, day into night, and life into death. These changes do not happen randomly but follow a prescribed pattern.

It is important to note that change from yin to yang and vice versa requires favorable internal conditions and favorable timing. For example, an egg changes into a chick with the application of heat only after the egg has been fertilized (applying heat to an unfertilized egg will not produce a chick). Next, change requires the right timing. The egg must be kept warm soon after it is fertilized and for a sufficient time afterward or the chick will not grow and hatch.

YIN-YANG BASICS

The ideas of yin and yang—combined with the concept of Qi—have been at the forefront of Chinese philosophy for centuries. It is a concept completely different from any Western philosophical thought.

Generally speaking, Western logic is based on opposition, which is the foundation of Aristotelian logic. According to this school of thought, contraries (such as "the table is square" and "the table is not square") cannot both be true. This philosophy has dominated Western thought for more than two thousand years.

The Chinese idea of yin-yang is completely different from this kind of thinking; yin and yang represent opposites, but at the same time they also complement each other. Every phenomenon can be itself and its contrary at the same time. On top of this, yin contains the root of yang and vice versa. So, contrary to Aristotelian logic, "A" can also be "non-A."

Every phenomenon in the multiverse is an interchange of cyclical movement, peaks and valleys. And the constant process of change through the interplay of yin and yang is the motivating force for all change and development. That means that yin and yang are always in a certain stage, degree of movement, or aggregation.

Yin and yang are two manifestations of the life force energy that flows within all living things. Said another way, yin and yang are flip sides of the same coin. This energy exists in substantial, tangible objects such as this book you are reading, your computer, and your body, as well as insubstantial, intangible things that you cannot see or hold, like scents and sounds, or even the process of sending a text message or email. Ancient Chinese philosophers referred to this life force energy as *Qi*, sometimes spelled chi, and pronounced *chee*.

The interaction of the energies of yin and yang explains how the universe operates, from its most simple to its most complex forms. When you understand yin-yang principles, you can improve your health, relationships, and spiritual well-being. This book will teach you all about the mysterious and intriguing energy foundation of the universe that will work to heal your neck and back pain while also improving your entire life!

THE ORIGINS OF YIN AND YANG

The theory of yin and yang grew from ancient Chinese peasants observing the cycles of day and night, summer and winter, growth and harvest. During the Warring States period from about 475 to 221 BC, the yin and yang school of philosophy emerged. Sages set out to interpret nature in a positive way and explain how to act in accordance with the laws of nature.

Yang, which corresponds to sky, was related to day, and yin, which corresponds to Earth, was related to night (as mentioned above). Thus, Heaven is considered yang, and the Earth, yin. Ancient Chinese people believed that Heaven was a round vault above a flat Earth. Therefore, yang is round and yin is square. Heaven contains the sun, moon, and stars, while Earth corresponds to space.

The original energy of the universe is incomprehensible. Some call it God, Oneness, or Universal Consciousness. Words can point to it but not fully describe It. There is no differentiation; everything is absolute, whole, and complete. It is beyond time and space and exhibits existence and nonexistence simultaneously. This nothingness was called *Wuji* by ancient Chinese philosophers. It is said that Wuji is the origin of the creation of Heaven and Earth.

The sun rises in the east (yang) and sets in the west (yin). If we face south, then east will be on the left and west on the right. In Chinese cosmology, compass directions were developed to be south facing.

Yin-yang philosophy believes that Qi is the life force that flows in all living entities. If Qi scatters and disperses, life ceases to exist and Qi takes on a different form. When Qi is collected and gathered, life emerges. The universe is abundant with Qi in many forms, from vaporous air to very dense matter. You can say that Qi is universal consciousness; even a rock has this consciousness of a sort because if it didn't, its atoms and molecules would disperse and it would dissolve into nothingness.

Qi wants to manifest its creative potential. This is what leads to the aspects of energy and matter.

Ancient philosophers believed that creation is the process by which undifferentiated nothingness, or Wuji, organizes into two apparent aspects. One of these is the unmanifest yang. Yang is active, moving and creating, and represents the immaterial, or intangible, state of Qi—that is, pure energy. The other is the manifest yin aspect, also referred to as matter or the material world. Yin represents the solid and static state of Qi. It is subtle and inactive.

■

Physicists recognize that matter and energy
are two forms of the same thing from Einstein's famous equation $E = mc^2$
(energy equals mass times the speed of light squared). According to yin
and yang, energy is yang and mass is yin.

■

YIN, YANG, AND YOUR BODY

The outside of the body is considered yang because yang is strong, hard, expansive, and superficial, protecting the delicate, soft, vital organs. Humans and animals are described as growing down from their heads to the Earth (yin). The left side of the body is considered masculine and its essence is the energy of Heaven (yang) that flows down to the (yin) Earth. Therefore, the right side of the body is yin and its energy flow is captured by the concept of a plant growing up from the Earth to the heavenly sky.

In the human body, Qi flows in this same cycle, down on the left side and up on the right. This is important when we seek to create balance.

Remember, disruption of Qi creates the dysfunction that eventually leads to chronic pain and inflammation. When going back to the root of our physical issues, we must address the causal elements of yin and yang energy flow and deal with any blockages or distortions of Qi. An example that illustrates this relationship is as follows: corresponding to yin and yang philosophy, the directional flow of fecal matter in the colon and intestines is up on the right and down on the left. So, to relieve constipation, you would massage the belly with your own hands circling clockwise to assist downward flow. For diarrhea, on the other hand, your hands would circle in a counterclockwise motion, increasing upward movement.

There are, however, times when organs are associated with the side of the body opposite them. For example, in acupuncture, if the Liver (located on the right side of the body) is being remedied, nine times out of ten the practitioner will needle the foot or the lower leg on the left side, opposite the organ. In addition, the left and right kidneys act opposite to the left and right sides of the body. The left Kidney is yin and the right Kidney is yang. The left Kidney is responsible for the cooling essence of the body, while the right Kidney is responsible for the heat that helps in transformation and circulation.

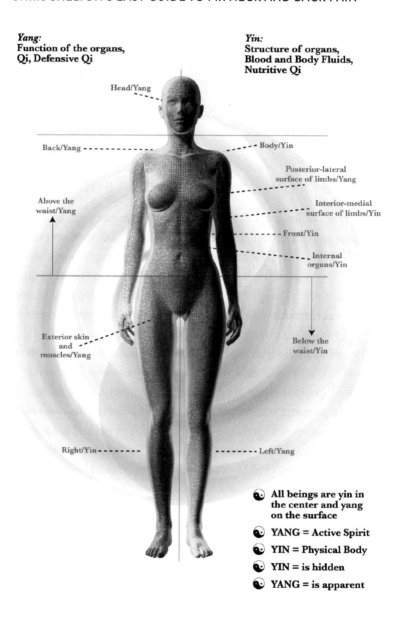

Yang:
Function of the organs, Qi, Defensive Qi

Yin:
Structure of organs, Blood and Body Fluids, Nutritive Qi

Head/Yang

Back/Yang

Body/Yin

Posterior-lateral surface of limbs/Yang

Above the waist/Yang

Interior-medial surface of limbs/Yin

Front/Yin

Internal organs/Yin

Exterior skin and muscles/Yang

Below the waist/Yin

Right/Yin

Left/Yang

All beings are yin in the center and yang on the surface

YANG = Active Spirit

YIN = Physical Body

YIN = is hidden

YANG = is apparent

LOCATIONS OF YIN AND YANG IN THE BODY

In classical Chinese medicine, physiology, typology, diagnosis, and remedy can all be understood as part of yin and yang philosophy (see figure above). Ultimately, the final aim is to balance and harmonize the yin and yang of the body. When the flow of these two forces is in harmony, wellness will result. It is also true that if one accumulates over the other or becomes deficient, the body will show signs of imbalance, disease, inflammation, and/or chronic pain.

To better understand and remedy yin and yang imbalances, it is helpful to know how to identify their areas within the body. Every part of the body is either yin or yang. Yin parts include the inferior, interior, and anterior, such as the feet, the internal organs, and the front of the body. Yang parts of the body are the superior, exterior, and posterior, such as the head, skin, and back. However, remember that yin and yang are *relative* concepts. For example, the abdomen would be considered yang relative to the legs because of its location above them. At the same time, the abdomen can be considered yin relative to the chest because of its location below. As a general rule, anything below another section of the body would be classified as yin relative to that section.

The exterior skin and muscles are considered yang because of their locations. Part of our immune system, also referred to as Defensive Qi, or Wei Qi, circulates in the skin and muscles. It functions to warm and moisten the interior organs. The inside of the body is yin. A disease considered to be yin is said to reach the nutritive level (digestive level) because nutritive Qi circulates within the internal organs.

The internal organs are also classified as yin and yang relative to each other. The yin organs are the Heart, Lungs, Spleen, Kidneys, and Liver, as well as the Pericardium (the sac enclosing the heart). Yang organs consist of the Small Intestine, Large Intestine, Stomach, Urinary Bladder, Gallbladder, and Triple Burner.

■

The Triple Burner is not an organ in Western medicine. In classical Chinese medicine, it corresponds to functions categorized into the Upper Burner, the Middle Burner, and the Lower Burner. It is like an information network that allows the internal organs to communicate with each other and ensure the proper functioning of each. The Triple Burner coordinates every function the organ performs.

■

In addition to being either yin or yang, each organ also contains elements of both. The structure of the organ and its blood, fluids, and essence relate to its yin aspect, while the functional activity and the motive force relate to the yang aspect of the organ. For example, although the Stomach is a yang organ, it also has functions of each aspect. Its yang function is rotting and ripening, while Stomach fluids and Stomach essence, including the ability to absorb nutrients, are yin aspects.

The back (including the back and outside of your arms, legs, and trunk) are where yang channels that protect your organs are located. Yin channels are located on the front (as well as on the inside of your arms and legs). These channels nourish the entire body.

As you can see, this is a detailed and nuanced system of delicate balance within the body. All aspects of yin and yang as well as their locations must be considered in order to effectively address the excess or deficiency of either one when the body displays symptoms of disease, pain, and/or inflammation.

UNDERSTANDING YIN AND YANG WITH DISEASE AND CHRONIC PAIN

Yin and yang are found throughout the body, from the tangible—like the structure of our internal organs, muscles, blood, and fluids—to the intangible, like our breath and the thoughts that flow throughout our day. If our constitution is vibrant, healthy, and strong, the body will have a natural way of restoring harmony when we have imbalances of yin and yang.

For example, if you had your gallbladder removed, the pancreas, spleen, and liver would pick up some of the functions and workload of the missing organ to achieve balance and harmony. I must emphasize that needing to have your gallbladder removed in the first place would have been caused by an imbalance of yin and/or yang that was not addressed. The body is remarkable in that it gives us symptoms and other signs of what's going on internally. If we can recognize these early and tend to their root causes, we can stop the progression of disease. It's when we let things go for too long that disease and chronic pain show up, including neck and back pain.

According to Chinese medicine, back and neck pain are considered a disease because it's an element of imbalance in the whole organism. One of the purposes of practicing Qigong is to allow you to become so aware of your body that you can help rectify a situation before it shows up as chronic pain or disease while at the same time balancing yin, yang, and the flow of Qi.

IN A NUTSHELL

Yin and yang principles explain how the universe was created from undifferentiated nothingness organized into two apparently opposite aspects—yin and yang. The principles also explain how the universe operates as a constantly changing cycle of relative yin and yang peaks and valleys. These same principles are used to explain the origins of disease (imbalances of yin and yang) and form the basis of remedy approaches. You can improve your life and health by balancing yin and yang in your body, mind, and spirit. When they are kept in balance, you will find that symptoms of disease, chronic pain, and inflammation fade away and no longer arise.

EVERYDAY TIPS
FOR BALANCING YIN AND YANG
FROM GRANDMASTER HUA CHING NI

Grandmaster Ni is a 38th-generation Chinese medicine and Taoist master. He started Yo San University in Los Angeles and the Tao of Wellness Center in Santa Monica. He has produced numerous books and videos on Taoist philosophy, Chinese medicine, and balanced living.

Here are his tips for balanced living:

- When time is gone, it is gone forever; be mindful of time.

- Enjoy your time on Earth and make it as wonderful as you can.

- Keep your household clutter-free daily to maximize free time.

- Prioritize: do the most difficult things first and finish what you've started.

- Break down larger projects into smaller, more achievable stages.

- Plan a reward for yourself after completing a particularly tough task.

- Include people who are important to you in your free time.

- Allow yourself to make mistakes. Worrying takes up too much time and energy.

▪ 3 ▪

THE FIVE ELEMENTS

The Five Elements are the cornerstone for everything I do in clinical practice, teach to the public, and apply to my own life. My intention in writing this book is to help you reverse neck and back pain, disease, and chronic pain. Disease prevention is based on the Five Elements, and finding equilibrium within them is essential when addressing pain and inflammation. Although this book's recommendations are specifically targeted for mending neck and back pain, incorporating a basic understanding of Five Element theory in your life will help you develop a greater awareness of your individual makeup and establish ways to stay in balance. In this chapter, we'll dive into the various expressions of these five phases of energy transformation to help you understand how important they are in maintaining your overall health and connection to the universe.

WHY THE FIVE ELEMENTS MATTER

The Five Elements (Wood, Fire, Earth, Water, and Metal), and specifically each person's dominant element, give us a deeper understanding of our unique selves. They describe our bodies and internal organs, our personality type, the way we think and perceive the world, our emotions, our virtues, the five aspects of spirit that make us individuals, the five sensory organs, the five areas of influence on the body . . . the list goes on and on.

They also reveal how our environment affects us, often without our even realizing it. This is important because with knowledge of the elements, we can respond appropriately when impacted by an external change or disruption.

There are many outside forces that can have a profound or subtle effect on us. For example, we are affected by the five seasons, and when those seasons are in discord with the body, disease may arise. (Most people think of four seasons, but in five-element principles the fifth season is the Indian summer months, when summer transitions into autumn.)

We are also affected by the five directions: north, south, east, west, and central. In addition, the five climatic conditions of wind, cold, heat, dampness, and dryness all have a tremendous impact on our personal element and our tendency toward balance or imbalance. We are further influenced by different flavors of food—sour, sweet or neutral (bland), salty, pungent or astringent, and bitter.

Just as the environment and weather surrounding a piece of wood or metal will have a specific impact on its form, what surrounds us will affect us in a unique way depending on our dominant element and state of balance or imbalance. Restoring equilibrium within requires knowledge of the Five Elements so that we can respond with the action most appropriate to our individual constitution.

Restorative actions can include many remedies, from diet to color therapy. Because each element can be impacted by an excess or a deficiency, signs of imbalance can often be easily resolved by incorporating or reducing variables specific to each.

Foods, when eaten in balance, can help the body. At the same time, cravings and/or aversion to one or more flavors can be an indicator of disease. We are influenced by the five colors (red/pink, green, blue/black, white/gray, and yellow/orange), and each can be added or removed from our wardrobe and our environment based on its emotional and psychological effects. We are further influenced by different patterns and textures. In fact, an aversion to or craving for certain patterns, textiles, textures, colors, and tastes can be an indicator of health issues as well as what is going on in the body. Once balance is restored between the elements within and around, one can begin to identify and gravitate toward those in harmony with their elemental makeup.

Along with each element's signs of imbalance come its tendencies toward negative emotions. Knowing more about our unique responses to external triggers can help us develop greater awareness so we can make choices and take actions that are in greater alignment with our true selves. We all need to take responsibility for our own growth and personal development. This growth arises from constant self-refinement and introspection, which help us achieve balance when it comes to emotions like hate, desire, shame, guilt, fear, sorrow, regret, and love, to name a few. Remember that these same negative emotions will eventually impact our organ health over time; taking steps to keep our dominant element in balance is a powerful preventative in keeping disease at bay.

Understanding how the Five Elements show up in our day-to-day lives will lead to a greater sense of well-being, health, and happiness overall. In addition, having a deeper understanding of the impact our external environment has on us can help us correct influences that adversely affect our judgment and ability to make sound decisions. Knowing that external pressures can cause you to deviate from your baseline of a naturally good and harmonious life (creating disease and discord in your life and possibly the lives of others) gives you the power to make positive changes.

Your stages of life are not determined by years but by your storehouse of energy. Years are only a mark of time. They don't actually represent your quality of life. Therefore, life's energy must be cultivated, nurtured, and treasured. This is the fundamental reason for understanding the Five Element cycles.

If you pay attention to the Five Element cycles, your internal and external energies will be harmonious. Your life will be longer and more fulfilling.

Self-adjustment, self-communion, self-discipline, self-government, self-knowledge, self-surrender, self-cultivation, self-control, self-examination, self-improvement, self-regulation, and self-sustenance allow you to understand the appropriate nature of things, within and without, and this keeps you in flow with all cycles. That is life.

YIN, YANG, AND THE FIVE ELEMENTS

In the previous chapter, you learned that yin and yang are in a constant state of flux and change, interdependent, always unfolding and developing. The Five Elements are simply an extension of yin and yang.

As yin and yang energies unfold, expanding from God/Tao/Universal Intelligence, they form the three treasures: Heaven, Earth, and human beings.

Yin-yang then continues to unfold into the four phases of energy: Wood, Fire, Metal, and Water. The harmonizing force for these four elements is the

Earth element. The inherent nature of the other four elements is to control or defeat one another.

In our bodies, the Earth element is represented by our Stomach and Spleen. The Stomach and Spleen are considered post-Heaven, or postnatal, Qi and are the origin of Qi and blood for the body. They are in the center of the body and are responsible for nourishing all other internal organs.

Healthy and strong digestion keeps our organs functioning properly and contributes to longevity. Even in our bodies, the Earth element holds all other elements together and acts as a lubricant, soothing the other four conflicting elements. The Earth element is considered a moderating or harmonizing force in the natural order of all things.

This is why proper digestion is a moderating force for all the other organs. The Earth element in nature helps keep the same balance. To maintain organ health, either as a preventative measure or in remedying symptoms of imbalance like neck and back pain, we must remember the importance of a healthy and strong digestive system and the role it plays in reestablishing and supporting greater health.

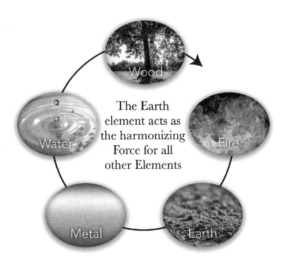

The Earth element acts as the harmonizing Force for all other Elements

THE CHARACTERISTICS OF THE FIVE ELEMENTS

Now that you've had some background on the importance of the Five Elements in both remedy and prevention of disease, let's spend some time learning more about them in greater detail.

Thousands of years ago, spiritually evolved ancients recognized that the evolution of the universe was not a linear process. They noted its polarization and organization into interrelated cyclical patterns, especially here on Earth.

Throughout history, other names have been used to describe the Five Elements. They've been called the Five Stages of Energy Transformation, the Five Phases of Energy Evolution, and the Wu-Hsing. *Wu* means "five" and *hsing,* used as a verb, means "to go through." Together, they can be translated as the five phases or the five passages. As in yin and yang theory, it's easy to get these principles confused, because they are also based on relativity and therefore may need to be interpreted in each unique circumstance.

People sometimes get tripped up by the names of the Five Elements. Don't take them literally. Instead, look at each element's characteristics as a way to understand what they're describing or symbolizing.

For example, the Wood element symbolizes the beginning of life, breaking through like a sprout from the Earth, awakening, generating. The energy of Wood also expresses upward movement. It is expansive and creative. It consumes and creates something new, like new plant growth in the spring that consumes the seed, water, and air to create its form. It encompasses the root of a sprout or the sprig of a tree or any plant pushing up to break through the soil.

The Wood element is also expressed by the sound of thunder breaking through thick clouds. As the first clap of thunder in the springtime has a way of awakening the animals and plants in hibernation, it also has a way of awakening us from delusion and our egocentric selves. Another example of Wood's presence is the expansive growth of a young, successful company that brings together the elements of a "recipe" for creative action or that combines different elements to form something new.

The Fire element symbolizes full growth, expanding life force, radiance, and beauty. The energy of Fire is represented as explosive and hot. It is a type of burning off. Fire speeds up the process of aging or becoming worn out; it consumes everything and destroys. It burns bright, then it burns out. Fire also has a way of beautifying whatever it touches. Examples of Fire energy are a bonfire, a firecracker, or an internal combustion engine. Emotionally, Fire shows up as untamed anger—quick, consuming, and explosive.

The Earth element is harmonizing, grounded, and nurturing. It is the root of prosperous growth and development. The energy represented by Earth is stability without being rigid. It is reliable and dependable, unmoving but not stagnant. It is a centered state of being.

One example of Earth energy is the foundation of a house. It upholds and supports the structure of a building, providing a safe environment. Another example would be the most responsible, stable person in a household, and a third, our physical bodies that provide a base for our thoughts, speech, and actions.

The Metal element represents collecting, reversing, retreating, and introverting. The energy of Metal is contracting and heavy. Its motion is inward and it is cold and stagnant. Examples of Metal energy include an overcast day in winter or water solidifying into ice. Emotionally, Metal shows up as depression, which is imploding and stagnant Liver energy.

The Water element is the reverting phase of contraction, collecting and regathering a new life force. It is invisible and waits for new breakthroughs. Water characteristics are fluid. They flow downward and are cool and liquid. It has a gathering and dispersing type of movement which can be either gentle and slow or quick, though not abrupt or sudden. For example, rainwater collecting in a container will trickle out quickly or slowly depending on the size of the filter or hole in the container. Think of the flow of a large crowd slowly filling a concert hall or football stadium, then rushing out after the show or the game is over. Another example is the breath of a person who is calm, slow, and gradual.

YIN AND YANG QUALITIES OF THE FIVE ELEMENTS

Each of the Five Elements has yin and yang states. The static state is yin and the dynamic state is yang. This is important in identifying the root energies and elements present when the body shows signs of imbalance. Both yin and yang have roles in the elements, and each will produce a unique expression. Without considering them as interacting forces, one might miss the subtleties of one or the other, and the opportunity to provide effective care will be limited.

The static and dynamic states of yin and yang can be found at every level of existence, from yearly cycles and seasons to each of the Five Elements within our bodies and in the seasons of our lives. The Five Elements are also present in our daily and monthly cycles and in the energy rotations between the internal organs of the body. The two systems of classification are interrelated and cannot be separated. Each element can therefore be looked at as also being either dynamic or static, yang or yin. See figure below.

Each element's manifestation changes quite drastically from state to state, demonstrating the polarity of expressions that are possible. Using nature as an example, we can see the dynamic (yang) aspect of the Wood element in climatic conditions like wind, snow, rain, thunder, and lightning, whereas the same element's static (yin) aspects are seen in trees, flowers, and all types of vegetation.

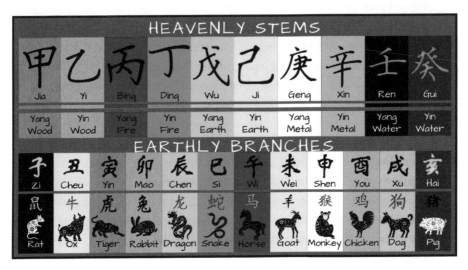

This variety of expression is further illustrated by the various forms taken by the Metal element. In its dynamic, or yang, state the Metal element is demonstrated by actions such as killing, battling, changing, and purifying, while its static, or yin, state includes such things as tools, instruments for harvesting the land, and weapons. You can see why all aspects must be considered when looking at each element. Viewing only one side could leave you without the whole picture of what is possible.

This relationship continues with the elements of Fire, Earth, and Water, as beautifully described by Grandmaster Ni:

> The dynamic aspect of yang Fire is the image of the life force expanding like a beautiful fire. In other words, the strong developing force is like the warmth of the sun's rays reaching the surface of the Earth. The yin aspect can be looked at like an image of a new life becoming fully grown or as one develops.

The dynamic aspect of yang Earth can be seen as the image of a luxuriant growth and prosperous development—stabilizing, neutral and strong. The yin aspect is an image of indistinguishable features and attributes or a weak stabilizing force.

The dynamic aspect of yang Water is an image of a life energy deeply within, like a pregnant mother nourishing the fetus. The yin aspect is the image of regathering of a new life force. Underground, like a seedling, waiting to sprout, invisibly, cultivating, and awaiting many breakthroughs.

—GRANDMASTER HUA CHING NI,
The Book of Changes and the Unchanging Truth

THE THREE CYCLES OF THE FIVE ELEMENTS

The Five Elements and yin and yang follow the same cycles as the rest of nature; these are the creative, controlling, and destructive cycles. Because we ourselves are a part of nature, these same cycles are present within us, and having a greater understanding of their functions and order can allow us to intervene with right timing when symptoms of disease set in. To begin with, I would like to share some of the underlying philosophy behind these elements and their cycles.

The first of the three cycles is the creative cycle, or generating sequence. This sequence describes the natural rise and decline of yin and yang. It is a simple system of the natural flow of energy in time and space, like the divisions of time during the day: morning to noon, noon to evening, evening to midnight, and so on. The creative cycle also describes the cycle of the moon and our life cycle, among others.

The first phase of the creative cycle begins with the Wood element, representing new growth. The second is the prospering phase and is related to Fire. The third phase is stabilizing, which is represented by the Earth element. The fourth phase is related to Metal and is when our energy starts to condense. The fifth and final phase relates to the Water element and is the time of decline and transformation into a new cycle.

The best way to remember the sequence is to first remember that the symbolic words Wood, Fire, Earth, Metal, and Water are just classifications or phases of the natural energy cycle. They are abstract representations of the cyclical nature of energy and the interwoven relationships of all phenomena, both seen and unseen. We sometimes refer to this sequence as the mother-child relationship. Water gives life to Wood, which creates vegetation. Wood gives life to Fire and Fire burns the Wood, creating ash that returns to the Earth. The Earth creates Metal as the mineral ore of the Earth and the Metal is transformed into liquid. We then repeat the cycle, starting with Water.

The creative cycle is considered a yang cycle, which moves in a clockwise direction. This cycle is a continuously flowing movement, with each phase leading into the next.

The next cycle is called the controlling cycle, or checking sequence. Each phase must control the others to keep their growth within reasonable limits. This cycle is also called the grandparent-child sequence because the "mother" element skips the "child" element and goes to the subsequent element. Wood controls Earth, the image of a sprout breaking though the earth. Earth controls Water, the image of earth damming water. Water controls Fire to keep the fire from blazing out of control. Fire controls Metal, the image of metal being melted for harvesting the land or engaging in battle.

The controlling cycle counterbalances the activity of the first sequence. It's considered a yin cycle, and it also moves in a clockwise direction. The controlling action occurs simultaneously and without pause. This constant transformation of one phase into another is what we call life. These transformations never cease as the universe creates itself perpetually. See figure below.

It is in this stage that the cycles will begin to show signs of discord in the human body. In terms of organ function, this controlling action is how the organs communicate with each other appropriately. However, if this sequence becomes excessive, it will create organ pathology or disease. For example, when we see conditions like gastroesophageal reflux disease (GERD), acid reflux, or heartburn, the common underlying cause (when observed from the perspective of the controlling cycle) is the Wood element (the Liver) overacting on the Earth element (the Spleen). This causes Qi to stagnate in the Stomach, not allowing it to descend the way it's supposed to. This, in turn, causes the Qi to rise upward, creating symptoms of imbalance.

Again, this cycle is designed to act as a check on the organs and only causes damage when it acts in excess. If the Heart overacts on the Lungs, it will dry them, causing symptoms such as dry cough, eczema, and asthma. If the Spleen overacts on the Kidneys, it will create dampness in the body and prevent the Kidneys' ability to excrete fluids. If the Lungs overact on the Liver, it can create excessive Liver heat, giving rise to abdominal distension and bloating. If the Kidneys are in excess, this will transfer to the Heart, causing edema and cold extremities.

The third cycle is called the destructive cycle, or the insulting sequence. This cycle is activated when the excess of one element results in the weakening or disturbance of another. This cycle moves in a counterclockwise direction. Fire destroys or extinguishes Water. Water floods the Earth and doesn't let Wood sprouts emerge. Wood is too hard for Metal to break through, and Metal can't be melted by Fire. See figure below.

The destructive cycle occurs when energies compete. This is how diseases develop. The following examples illustrate some common symptoms of disease that result once this cycle is initiated within organs in the body:

- If Liver Qi attacks the Lungs, this will cause Liver Qi to stagnate and move upward, obstructing the chest and affecting breathing, possibly causing asthma.

- If Heart Qi attacks the Kidneys, this can affect the excretion function of the Kidneys, causing conditions such as night sweats, restless legs syndrome, and nocturnal emissions.

- If Spleen Qi attacks the Liver, this will inhibit the Liver's function of moving Qi and blood, which will then cause symptoms such as tiredness, menstrual irregularities, and digestive issues.

- If Lung Qi attacks the Heart, this will create phlegm, which will appear as poor circulation of the Heart's Qi, causing symptoms such as mental restlessness, forgetfulness, and brain fog.

- If Kidney Qi attacks the Spleen and the Kidneys can't transform the fluids, symptoms of phlegm, fibroids, and digestive issues may result.

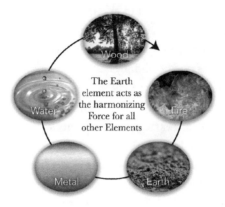

Creative Cycle

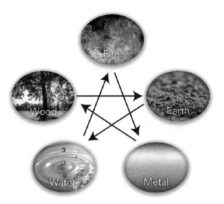

Controlling Cycle

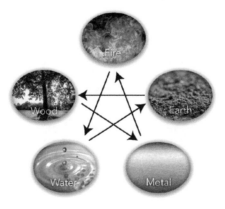

Destructive Cycle

If you study these three cycles of the Five Elements, you will gain a deeper understanding of how disease shows up in the body. Using the Five Element system, we can better understand and assess what is going on and develop helpful strategies to combat disease based on the knowledge of functional interactions between internal organs.

You can discover and begin to recognize what it looks like when any (or all) of the organs are out of balance or are not communicating with other organs in the proper sequence. When we combine the Five Elements with family structure, environmental factors, diet, and climatic conditions, we can come up with a very effective means for understanding disease and chronic pain, how to rectify it, and, most importantly, how to prevent it. This same understanding is what underlies the remedies found in this book to relieve neck and back pain.

To incorporate this deep investigation into the energies present in the body, we use all the tools that we have access to—for example, taking the pulse, looking at the tongue, and reading the face, as well as using the five assessments that include listening, palpating/touching, smelling, looking, and asking. All these methods allow us to see how the outside environment is affecting the inside environment and how the inside environment is showing signs of imbalance or disease.

Interestingly, Five Elements philosophy is so expansive that it can even be used in military strategy, as in the book *The Art of War*. In addition, feng shui, nutrition, herbology, pharmacology, astrology, farming, government, family, and business structures can also be viewed as extensions of the Five Elements.

The Five Elements and natural law are the foundations of the appropriate way to live one's life. The chaos we see in the political arena, our homes, family lives, and within ourselves can be seen as evidence that the Five Elements are out of balance.

This law is not man's law; it is universal law. When we are attuned, we can see the appropriateness in all situations and avoid unnecessary calamities within ourselves, our community, and the world that we live in. By striving to maintain this harmony within and without, we will find that physical symptoms of imbalance arise less frequently and when they do, we will be able to respond effectively, restoring ease and flow.

PERSONALITY TYPES AND THE FIVE ELEMENTS

To deepen your understanding of the Five Elements and the influence they have, it is both helpful and interesting to see how they show up in the deepest parts of your being, including your personality. Everyone has a dominant personality element (Wood, Fire, Earth, Water, Metal) that shapes who they are, how they interact with the world, and which diseases they're more likely to attract when out of balance. Unique personality traits, like being shy, talkative, funny, or serious, correspond to different strengths and weaknesses of one's element, which also point to potential health risks and imbalances.

The Five Element Questionnaire is one of the major assessment, diagnostic, and remedy tools that I use. I have combined what I know from ancient Chinese medicine with my many years of clinical practice to create a targeted list of questions that will reveal your individual makeup. When you discover your dominant element as well as your weakest one, you will be able to adopt and integrate empowering ways to think, eat, and live. You will also begin to honor and recognize your true nature to a greater extent while moving away from inauthentic expressions of self.

So if you haven't done it yet, take the Five Element Questionnaire by scanning the QR code below or visiting www.chrissheltonseasyguide.com.

You will discover your unique typology made up of your primary, secondary, and weakest elements along with the organ systems they rule.

Keep in mind that when you deviate from your primary typology, it's a marker for potential disease. For example, a Wood type is ideally creative or in a managerial position. If a Wood type has an aversion to conflict and doesn't want to use his or her voice to speak up when appropriate, this is a deviation from typology and can contribute to many types of imbalance, including Liver dysfunction and depression. Once imbalance sets in, there is a domino effect. When assessing the pathway of physical discomfort, like neck and back pain, we see first that minor symptoms arise as early signals. Learning the subtleties of elements present in our bodies so that even the slightest change can be detected early on gives us the opportunity to reestablish harmony and find the health and vitality we are searching for.

CHINESE FACE READING AND THE FIVE ELEMENTS

What's really fun about Chinese face reading is that after studying it, you can look at somebody and understand their personality, the way they think, and their past traumas simply by recognizing certain features and patterns in the face. Chinese face reading gives the practitioner a window deep into what's really going on beneath the surface. It is an ancient diagnostic tool that remains unparalleled, especially when dealing with hard-to-treat or chronic issues.

Face reading was developed thousands of years ago because Chinese doctors didn't think it was appropriate to touch women in order to diagnose them. They had to come up with another method. The practice was a sound, reliable way to understand the physiology, psychology, and pathology of a person as well as potential illnesses. Today, face reading is still a valuable tool to help us understand our own typology and when we're deviating from it.

Most people who take my face-reading classes are not in the medical field. Rather, they are lawyers, HR people, or those looking to find their soulmate—people who want to better understand human nature. The shape and features of someone's face tell us what element type the person is and can open up a world of information.

Face reading goes much deeper than simply understanding one's personality, as in the Enneagram, for example. Once you become adept at the practice of face reading, you'll begin to discover how to rectify any deviations you notice with the various tools you'll find in this book.

By looking at the shape of someone's face, you can determine their dominant element. A Wood type will have either a rectangular or inverted-trapezoid-shaped face. A triangular or heart-shaped face belongs to the Fire type while an Earth person will have a square or trapezoid-shaped face. An oval or diamond-shaped face indicates a Metal typology, whereas a face with a circular shape is characteristic of a Water type.

If you look at a person's face or look in the mirror, you will see that the left and right sides do not usually align. This is because what people feel on the inside is not necessarily what they project to the world. Oftentimes, people suffering with symptoms of disease do not know themselves sufficiently to understand what is truly going on, let alone share their vulnerabilities and deep traumas. It takes eyes of wisdom to read the language of the body and soul. This ancient practice is key.

Yin and yang aspects are also shown on the face. The right side of the face is yin and reflects how we want to be perceived in public or by others. The left side of the face is yang and is our internal self. This side of the face is private and shows how we truly are on the inside.

Even though each of us has a primary element typology, different parts of the face also represent the various elements and organs. Therefore, facial examination allows the practitioner to get an in-depth look at the internal state of the body.

The Wood element shows up on the eyebrows, brow bone, jaw, and temples. The Fire element appears in the glistening of the eyes and the tips and corners of the nose, lips, ears, eyebrows, chin, etc. The Earth element shows up in the lower cheeks, the mouth, and the lips, whereas the Metal element can be seen on the nose, cheekbones, cheeks, and skin. The Water element is most visible under the eye area and on the ears, chin, and philtrum (the vertical groove on the upper lip).

We take everything into consideration when assessing the health of an individual (or ourselves). Every line, every feature on your face, the size and location of those features, and any markings tell us how you think and, on a deeper level, what traumas you've been through. Most importantly, they expose what potential diseases are lurking inside your body. The face becomes a map we can follow, showing us the starting place of current imbalance and the path it has taken. Face reading reveals the secrets of the body and mind so that we can fully understand someone and address the deepest causes of their pain, inflammation, and disease in a more effective and complete way.

Chinese face reading is a fascinating diagnostic tool. When I see clients in the clinic, besides taking their pulse and looking at their tongue, I read their face, and I find that the face is most telling when it comes to long-term emotional events and potential diseases. If you'd like more information on Chinese face reading, I recommend Lillian Bridges' book *Face Reading in*

Chinese Medicine. Besides being helpful for understanding yourself at a deeper level, it's useful for business and personal relationships.

ENERGETICS AND YOUR TYPOLOGY

The most important takeaway from this book is understanding your element typology and the implications of deviations from it.

When you digress from your true self based on the Five Elements, it indicates possible diseases that may arise as well as chronic pain and illness you might be dealing with in the present and/or future. By comprehending this, you will also begin to understand diseases or problems that you have had in the past.

Scan the QR code below for a list taken from a workshop that I did with Dr. Mao Shing Ni at Yo San University in 2019. The list is quite detailed. Dr. Mao also listed reflections and questions that people with specific typologies might ask themselves, helping to uncover traits, key points, and actions that they should be engaged in to stay in balance.

4

HOW WE GET SICK

The book *The Yellow Emperor's Classic of Medicine: A Translation of Huangdi Neijing Suwen with Commentary* by Mao Shing Ni says it best: "To prevent illness after disease sets in is like digging a well after one has become thirsty; or forging one's weapons after one is engaged in battle . . . wouldn't that be too late?"

Before we dive deep into what creates neck and back issues, let's talk about how we get sick because these topics are related. Remember that when the whole body is aligned and in balance, sickness and disease will subside. Even a common cold is a signal that there is work to be done, and remedying imbalance when it sets in, even on a small scale, will eventually bring greater overall health to all interrelated parts of the body.

What are the root causes of illness and what can we do to prevent getting sick? According to Chinese medicine, how we get sick, or our susceptibility to illness, is based on our overall constitution.

What does this mean? At the time of conception, your environment predetermines the "battery" of your life; this battery is rooted in the Kidneys. Your overall environment includes God or the universe (whatever you prefer to call it), your parents, or genetics, and the immediate environment you were born into. Your Kidney Qi predetermines how long your life will be—unless you get hit by a car or die prematurely from some disease or severe illness.

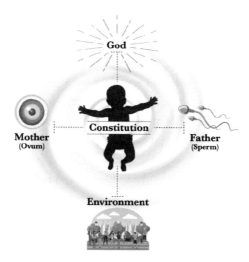

We can tell the strength of someone's Kidneys by looking at the size of their ears, philtrum, and chin. The bigger your ears are, the stronger your chin, and the longer or deeper your philtrum, the more robust your Kidney well will be. (A Kidney well is to the body what capacity is to a battery.) These traits demonstrate that the genetic Qi, also known as Upright Qi, is very strong.

If somebody has smaller ears, a smaller or recessed chin, and a small philtrum, they will tend to fight off stress or illness poorly. You may know someone—maybe even yourself—who has smaller ears. If you went out and got a couple of drinks with friends, you might not recover quite as well as your friends with larger ears. Why? Because your Kidney well is not as strong as theirs.

This means that we have to preserve this Kidney Qi, our constitutional Qi, and really understand and accept the fact that our own constitution might be a little weaker than those of others. There is hope when we focus on what we can do to strengthen it because we're all different. Any positive changes will impact the total health of our body and its ability to ward off pain and disease.

Let's start with the most important thing first.

STRATEGIES FOR PRESERVING QI

Maintaining a healthy and robust constitution is paramount in healing and preventing further neck and back pain. If you know you have a weaker constitution, the number one thing you need to do to preserve your Kidney Qi is get enough sleep. Sleep is critical in helping to preserve health and longevity, and taking 20- or 30-minute power naps every day is beneficial for good health. It can add years to your life. If the body has a large reservoir of energy, you will find that it responds with greater resiliency in stressful situations. This is an essential step toward keeping chronic neck and back pain at bay.

So if you have a less robust constitution, take time to listen to your body: if you tend to burn the candle at both ends, find yourself being overwhelmed by stress very easily, and/or you seem to get sick often, recharge by getting additional rest.

Another thing that will enhance Kidney Qi and help your overall constitution is practicing Qigong and Tai Chi, which have historically been known as the "fountain of youth." These practices focus on the lower Tan Tien region, one of three major energy centers in the body, which is connected to the Kidneys (our batteries). As we age, this battery naturally declines. Practices like Qigong help preserve Kidney Qi and slow down the aging process, creating strong bones and allowing the muscles of the body to maintain greater elasticity and durability.

As stated earlier, Qigong also gives us tools to process and release our emotions, which are causal factors in creating imbalances that lead to dysfunction and disease. When toxic emotions are processed and released from the body, they will not be stored by the organs and tissues of the system, and this eliminates the underlying causes of disease, chronic pain, and inflammation.

So when considering things we can do to build our overall constitution, sleep is number one and practices like Qigong and Tai Chi are number two.

DIET AND NUTRITION

The next thing that we have to look at is what we're putting into our bodies.

Our body is a complete system that operates as a whole. And like any system, what you put into it is what you get. Toxic input generates toxic output. If we want our body to operate at full capacity, we need to make sure we are providing the right fuel for it to do so. If we want the bones, muscles, and tissues to be healthy and strong, we must provide the body with the nutrients it needs to build them effectively.

Let's start with genetically modified and processed foods. I've heard various arguments, like the one that says there's no scientific proof that genetically modified foods actually create disease in the body. I believe that anything that goes against nature, or natural law, is not good for us. If you have a stronger constitution, you may not see the ramifications, or ill effects, of eating modified or processed foods for quite some time. I know many people who look fit but eat a lot of fast food instead of food that is cooked at home—food that's organic and wholesome, prepared with love and positive intentions. Some may not see the consequences right away because their constitutions are stronger, but over time they will weaken their own DNA, and this will affect future generations. You may not see the full damage of an unhealthy diet in your lifetime, but if you have kids and grandkids, the effects of genetically modified and processed foods may show up later in the family chain.

I found this to be true for myself. My mother did not take good care of herself when she was pregnant with me. She ate a lot of processed foods along with several over-the-counter medications. Even after I was able to eat solids, my diet was not wholesome. It was filled with a lot of unhealthy, processed foods like hot dogs, cheese, and milk. As a result, I was often sick as a baby and a young child. I suffered from convulsions, breathing issues, and rare skin diseases. I was even studied by doctors at Stanford Hospital. Luckily for me, I had a strong constitution. Over many years, through making both minor and major changes, I was able to regain my health.

Dr. Francis M. Pottenger wrote a report years ago on a phenomenon called the Pottenger Cat Study. He conducted a study on cats between 1932 and 1942 by dividing them into two groups. Those in Group A were fed a diet of two-thirds raw meat, one-third raw milk, and cod-liver oil. Group B was fed a diet of two-thirds *cooked* meat, one-third raw milk, and cod-liver oil. He first noticed that the fecal matter from Group B, those eating cooked meat, was unhealthy. The vegetation died in the area surrounding where he dumped the cats' feces, but the feces from cats eating foods natural to their environment didn't have that effect. He also found that with each generation, the cats fed cooked meat (which is not natural for them) were sickly. By the third generation, they were no longer able to reproduce; they became sterile, and their family trees died out.

Always remember that food is not only fuel, it is also medicine. The unhealthy foods that we eat don't always show up in our constitution right away, but we will notice the consequences eventually.

So how should you eat?

Make sure the foods that you eat are wholesome. Most of your vegetables should be blanched (briefly immersed in boiling water) or lightly sautéed.

Try to avoid cold and raw foods because they can disrupt digestion. It is also important to avoid foods that trigger inflammation, especially sugar (the main culprit). Alcohol is also highly inflammatory, especially when used in excess. If you like to enjoy a glass of wine at night, that's fine as long as it doesn't negatively impact your health. Talk to your primary care physician to make sure it's okay.

Excessive consumption of alcohol and foods that are greasy, fatty, fried, processed, or genetically modified invites the possibility of disease, especially if you have a weak constitution.

How you eat is also important. If you sit in front of the TV set, if you're mindless while you eat, or if your family has disagreements and arguments at the dinner table, that will also cause inflammation in the body. It will disrupt your digestive system and create the potential for disease. The same applies to standing while eating, eating on the run, and not chewing your food thoroughly.

Paying attention to how and what we eat is also important because the stomach controls what we refer to as our "Qi thoroughfare," or our "post-Heaven Qi," as opposed to the Jing Qi, or our "pre-Heaven essence" that we are born with. The post-Heaven Qi is what we create in our lives through proper diet and nutrition.

The bottom line is that healthy digestion is not just about the food you eat. The Earth element, which energizes the Stomach and Spleen, acts as a harmonizing force for all internal organs. Therefore, it's essential to take care of your Stomach to keep the body's organs functioning properly. Remember, imbalances of the body and its tissues have their origin in organ dysfunction. Thus, we can impact chronic pain and inflammation by keeping our organs in balance. Because the Stomach plays such a central role in the entire system, it is essential to follow these guidelines:

- Eat foods that are healthy, and eat mindfully.

- Avoid heated discussions around mealtimes, at night, or before the kids go to school for the day. Choose a time that is appropriate.

- Take extra care of yourself if you live in an abusive environment or a household where there is frequent bickering, arguing, or high levels of stress.

- Don't eat on the run. Minimize fast food and eating out. Both activities will contribute to the degeneration of the body and will cause you to get sick.

Healthy habits enable the digestive system to do what it's supposed to do—move smoothly and evenly to assist in the proper functioning of all organs.

HYDRATION

It is imperative for the ultimate health of our bodies to hydrate ourselves properly by drinking plenty of room-temperature water. Since water makes up 79 percent of our muscles, 90 percent of our blood, and 60 percent of our entire body, staying hydrated is a necessary part of staying healthy.

Sufficient hydration protects the spinal cord, tissues, and joints. Furthermore, water helps maintain the balance of bodily fluids for functions like digestion, absorption, and the creation of saliva. It also helps maintain organ function, especially kidney function (our storehouse of energy). Also, drinking room-temperature water in place of soda or other sugary drinks can assist in weight loss.

It is important to be aware that drinking too much water can create blood deficiencies and contribute to anemia. According to the US National Academies of Sciences, Engineering, and Medicine, there is no exact amount of water that should be consumed daily. The amount will depend on each individual's constitution and how active they are. However, as an average, the daily intake for men should be around 125 ounces (15.5 cups), and women may need closer to 91 ounces (11 cups). About 80 percent of the water we consume should come from drinks, including water, and the rest from foods like fresh fruits and vegetables.

YOUR DNA

Next up is genetics. In addition to our pre-Heaven essence (the Qi we were born with), our genetics determine how strong our constitution will be and our propensity for disease. It is important to remember, however, that people are not doomed to their genetics. Science is now proving that even when someone is genetically predisposed to or has a family history of heart disease, diabetes, or migraines, they will avoid disease if they change what they eat, their environment, and how they respond to stressful situations.

And what's really cool is that science is now proving that if we go back 32 or 33 generations and see that the DNA helix itself has strands prone to, say, heart disease, your DNA still *wants* to be healthy. In 2015, Deepak Chopra and Rudolph E. Tanzi, PhD, outlined these discoveries in their book *Super Genes*. What's fascinating and enlightening about their work is that it shows us that we have some control over—and even play a major part in—transforming our health.

In clinical practice, when I see people with diseases that they've had a long time—even a degeneration of the nervous system or a degenerated disc—my attitude is that sometimes people's bodies get stuck and they need someone like me to come along and facilitate the body's own healing process. Your DNA *wants* to be healthy. Your body does not want to be sick. It's always looking for a way to achieve balance, just like our environment is. In the outside world, certain weather conditions seem abnormal. We experience natural disasters that are horrifying, but they're actually the Earth and nature's way of trying to restore harmony and balance. We are an extension of nature, and our bodies are no different.

Back and neck pain are signals that the body is in need of restored balance. Whether you have a weaker constitution or there are genetic factors involved in your specific circumstance, you assist the body in finding the equilibrium it seeks when you begin to make healthy choices.

SETTING HEALTHY BOUNDARIES

According to the ancient principles of Chinese medicine and Qigong, physical health is a byproduct of emotional health. Therefore, when you take care to create a healthy emotional environment, you will find that your overall physical state improves.

How do you begin to create a healthy emotional environment? Surround yourself with people who are supportive and loving and who respect your boundaries. People who talk negatively to you or who aren't uplifting you, your cause, or your life's purpose don't need to be in your life. There are plenty of people out there with the same vibration as you. Align yourself with them instead.

Unfortunately, most people are wrapped up in their own egos. They don't know that they're sick or toxic and that they're projecting those toxins onto you. Their negativity can create illness within you if you're not careful. Understand that and recognize it so you can take steps to protect yourself.

There is an amazing book called *How to Suffer in 10 Easy Steps: Discover, Embrace and Own the Mechanics of Misery* by William Arntz. In one of the chapters, Arntz describes how each of us has a worldview, or paradigm—a way of viewing the world based on our life experiences, wisdom, and the knowledge we've gained so far. He points out that many times people will try to change or alter your worldview, especially if they feel threatened by it. Challenging you gives them a false sense of power or superiority. So pay attention to who you hang around with.

You can be eating right, your constitution can be strong, and you can have a strong spiritual connection, but if you're around people that are toxic and sick, then guess what? That will make you sick too. What can you do?

First and foremost, protect yourself by creating healthy relationships and maintaining healthy boundaries. I love Cesar Millan, the Dog Whisperer, because he says that like dogs, people need boundaries, rules, and limitations. I agree with him.

So set healthy boundaries, eat healthy food, and really pay attention to your environment, including who is in it. Everyone's a snowflake; we each need to figure out what's uniquely right for us. I recommend reading the books listed in appendix 2 as well as *The Tao of Nutrition* by Dr. Mao Shing Ni, which discusses the energetic properties of food along with indications and contraindications and gives some simple recipes to enhance your health and change the trajectory of disease.

HOW EMOTIONS AFFECT QI

Emotional stress upsets the smooth flow of Qi (ascending/descending, entering/exiting). This disruption leads to stagnation, which can eventually lead to blood stasis, especially in women and specifically concerning anger and guilt. Qi stagnation can also lead to heat, dampness, and phlegm, affecting the Liver, Lungs, and Heart. All emotions affect the Heart indirectly because the Heart houses the Mind. A tongue with a red tip is commonly seen in those with emotional problems related to the

Heart, although the effect on any given organ depends on whether the emotion is expressed or repressed.

The Minister of Fire (the fire of the Kidneys, or our motive force) is stirred by emotional stress. Stress creates heat and an upward movement of Qi that disturbs the Heart and Pericardium. This may lead to the following symptoms:

Full Heat — Feeling hot, excessive thirst, dry mouth, insomnia, mental restlessness, red face, manic behavior, hyperactivity, anxiety, or a red tongue with a red tip and yellow coating.

Empty Heat — (If a person is yin deficient): Feeling hot at night, dry mouth with a desire to drink in small sips, malar (cheek) flush, insomnia, manic behavior, mental restlessness, fidgetiness, anxiety, having a red tongue with a red tip without a coating.

Yin Fire — (If there is heat in the upper chest and head): Red face, thirst, feeling hot in the face, depression, anxiety, having a red tip on the tongue. (If there is cold below the chest): Cold feet, feeling cold, pale tongue.

The Pericardium also houses the Mind and is affected by emotions. It is responsible for "movement" toward others (that is, sociability, love, and family relationships). It is related to the Liver in the Yin Linking Vessel, an internal vessel that controls the interior of the body. Many Pericardium points have a deep influence on your mental state, and by gently massaging specific points, you can help relieve yourself of many types of emotional problems.

The Yin Linking Vessel links all the yin acupuncture meridians and helps remove blockages, specifically in the Liver, Spleen, and Kidneys. It also communicates with the conception channel and helps store excess Qi when there is a shortage. The conception channel is the meridian that flows through the front, center midline of the body. See Yin Linking Vessel figure on the next page.

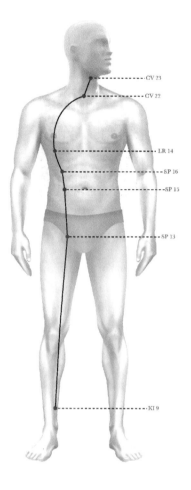

Pericardium 6 (PC 6) is an acupuncture point that lifts mood and eases depression; adding this point to any other increases the therapeutic effect. It is a connecting point of the Pericardium channel (as shown in the figure to the right), so it connects to the Triple Burner. Pericardium 7 calms the mind and settles anxiety, and Pericardium 5 helps with mental confusion.

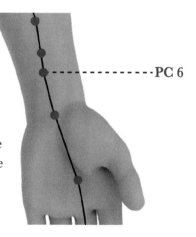

For more details on acupuncture points, download your Location and Function of Acupoints to Relieve Back Pain guide by scanning the QR code below or visit: www.chrissheltoneasyguide.com.

MENTAL AND EMOTIONAL HEALTH

The number one cause of premature death and disease is emotional stress and trauma. We all have emotional baggage—some of us more and some less. Disease shows up when we don't express our emotions appropriately and they become stored in the organs of the body, creating toxic effects with widespread consequences.

That means you have to learn to check in with yourself regularly. Ask yourself, "Is this bothering me? Do I need to say something or do I need to let it go?" Or "Do I need to *not* say something but still let it go?" Some of the worst diseases I have seen occur when a person is in total ignorance of their emotional state.

The English word "emotion" does not capture the Chinese view of the emotional causes of disease and imbalance. In Western terminology, *emotion* includes positive feelings, like hope and joy. That's not what I'm talking about. I'm referring to emotions that are associated with mental suffering as the cause of disease. When suffering takes over our minds and therefore possesses us, disease results.

However, emotions become the cause of disease only when they are long-standing or very intense. It is not each instance of a negative emotion that has long-term consequences; it is the negative emotion repeated frequently over a long period of time or at a high intensity that creates the most damage.

Each emotion is associated with a particular yin organ that has a reciprocal function in the body, meaning that when it is positively or negatively affected, so is the part of the body that works opposite to it that keeps it in balance.

Each organ also has a psychic energy that turns into a negative emotion when triggered by external circumstances. Emotional stress injures the organ, and the resulting organ disharmony causes further emotional, and later physical, imbalance. With Qigong, these harmful emotions can be released from the organs of the body, eliminating unfavorable long-term effects.

To recap: like all imbalance and disease, neck and back pain are rooted in organ dysfunction that is activated by negative emotions that become stored in the body. Therefore, the health of our bodily tissues is in direct proportion to our emotional well-being.

Let's take a closer look at these causal emotions as well as their positive counterparts, which can arise once the negative aspects are released. The nuances are important to be aware of when investigating emotional roots of physical imbalance. The closer we get to identifying the true underlying emotional traumas stored deep within our organs, the greater capacity there will be to facilitate their release and initiate healing. Also, by better understanding any associated symptoms you are experiencing (in addition to your neck and back pain), you will get a bigger picture of how to address the root causes.

ANGER

Anger is one of the biggest contributors to disease in the body. Not because anger is bad, but because people often don't express it properly. Suppressed anger creates conditions like depression, trigeminal neuralgia, neurological issues, migraines, and all sorts of digestion disorders including Crohn's disease, colitis, irritable bowel syndrome (IBS), and menstrual problems. That's right—if you have menstrual or premenstrual symptoms, it's considered a disease in Chinese medicine! So look at what is going on in your life. What's making you angry, and how are you holding on to it?

Anger is not a "bad" emotion. It is there to help us create positive change in the world. But if your anger is causing depression, overeating, or substance abuse, or if it's causing you to go home and kick the dog or cat or get in a fight with your spouse and kids, then you know that it is no longer serving you. Simple practices like Qigong and Tai Chi are excellent ways to help you manage anger as well as the unwanted side effects of such a powerful emotion.

I talk about anger a lot, but it can often mask other negative emotions as well. That is, sometimes people are angry because they're covering up a more vulnerable feeling. For example, if you're afraid, you may cover up that fear with anger. If you're sad and don't want to show it, you may express yourself with anger instead. Although it's masked in sadness, even long-standing depression may be due to repressed anger or resentment, often harbored toward a family member.

It's important to be aware of the other emotions associated with an accumulation of anger. These include resentment, feeling aggrieved, frustration, irritation, rage, indignation, animosity, and bitterness. If anger is bottled up, it causes stagnant Liver Qi or Liver Blood stasis. If anger is expressed, it causes Liver Yang or Liver Fire Blazing. Only when anger is observed and released can it pass through the body in a neutral way.

Anger makes Qi rise, so symptoms will manifest in the head and neck. In addition to general pain and inflammation, these symptoms may include headaches, tinnitus, dizziness, red face, thirst, a bitter taste in the mouth, or a red tongue with red sides.

Under the influence of anger, the pulse will be full and wiry in all positions, meaning that on both the right and left wrists it will feel like a wire under your fingertips. The tongue will be red with even redder sides and will have a dry, yellow coating. Liver Qi can invade the Stomach if someone gets angry at mealtimes or the Intestines if a person gets angry one or two hours after eating. Anger also affects the Heart. If anger has caused stagnant Liver Qi, expressing it can be a helpful first step in eventually releasing it.

The positive counterparts to anger are power, dynamism, creativity, and generosity. By practicing healthy habits regarding feelings of anger, we can positively impact our Liver Qi. The Liver is related to the Gallbladder, which is the source of courage to make important decisions and change one's life. If Liver Blood is deficient, there is fear; if it's abundant, a person is fearless and decisive. By practicing Qigong and allowing anger to flow through us without becoming stored in our organs, we can benefit from the more balanced expressions of this energy.

JOY

Joy as a cause of disease suggests an excessive craving for mental excitement—also known as a life of "work hard, play hard." An excessive amount of joy injures the Heart and makes it larger. Symptoms include palpitations, insomnia, restlessness, talking a lot, red tip of the tongue, pulse overflowing (feeling too strong against your fingertip when gently pressed), and pulse being empty in Heart position (feeling like a half-empty balloon when gently pressed, especially when taking the pulse on the left wrist at the crease in the base of the palm). A migraine that comes on after receiving good news, a sudden burst of laughter triggering a heart attack, and overexcitement leading to tears in children are all examples of too much joy. When joy is in balance, one will feel calm and experience clear thinking and sound judgment.

WORRY

Today's modern society fosters insecurity, and worry is a constant companion. Many people are tense. They do everything in a hurry and are always pressed for time. Worry knots Qi, causes Qi stagnation, and negatively affects the Lungs and Spleen.

Worry may also affect the Liver directly, causing Liver Qi stagnation or Liver Yang Rising. This affects the shoulders, producing pronounced stiffness and aching at the trapezius muscles (on the tops of the shoulders). When worry affects the Lungs, symptoms include an uncomfortable feeling in the chest, slight breathlessness, tense shoulders, a dry cough, a pale complexion, and a tight or wiry Lung pulse (found below the right wrist crease on the radial artery). When worry affects the Spleen, symptoms will include poor appetite, epigastric discomfort, abdominal pain and distension, tiredness, a pale complexion, and a tight, weak Spleen pulse. Worry also affects the Heart (like all emotions do), causing Heart Qi stagnation, palpitations, a tight chest, and insomnia.

The positive emotional counterpart to worry is Spleen Qi's capacity for concentration, focus, and memorization. Once the trapped energy of worry is released, the mind can use it in powerful ways.

PENSIVENESS

Similar to worry, this emotion includes brooding, constantly thinking about certain events or people, nostalgic hankering for the past, thinking intensely about life, and excessive mental work. In extreme cases, pensiveness can lead to obsessive thoughts. Pensiveness affects the Spleen and also knots Qi. It causes symptoms similar to those for worry but is limited to the Spleen.

The positive counterpart to pensiveness is quiet contemplation and meditation. Releasing excessive mental energy through Qigong and Tai Chi allows one to quiet the mind.

SADNESS AND GRIEF

Sadness and grief are some of the more painful emotions that can easily accumulate in the body. This category includes regret for actions taken or decisions made in the past. Western people who regret the dissolving of their past relationships or marriages are often more prone to neck pain.

Sadness and grief primarily affect the Heart, but the Lungs also suffer because both are close together in what is referred to as the Upper Burner. Extending from the mouth to the stomach, this region takes in air, liquid, and solids and is also responsible for harmonizing the Heart and Lungs. Some Chinese doctors believe that unexpressed grief, borne without tears, can affect the Kidneys. In addition, sadness and grief from widowhood, divorce, the death of a child, or a relationship breakup can manifest as breast lumps and cancer.

Sadness and grief deplete Qi and after some time lead to Qi stagnation. Symptoms include a pale complexion, a weak voice, tiredness, crying, shortness of breath, and a feeling of compression in the chest. In addition, women often experience blood deficiency and abnormal menstruation.

FEAR

The intensity of fear has a strong impact on the body and directly affects our ability to engage with life. Fear includes chronic fear, anxiety, and sudden fright. This emotion depletes Kidney Qi and causes stagnation in the Upper Burner. If the Heart is strong, Qi will descend, possibly resulting in incontinence or diarrhea. If the Heart is weak, Qi will rise in the form of Empty Heat (for example, palpitations, insomnia, or dry mouth); this is especially common in older people and women. Liver Blood and Gallbladder deficiencies are also indicated with fear.

The positive counterparts that arise when fear is in balance are flexibility, yielding in the face of adversity, and a quiet endurance of hardship. Once the negative emotion of fear is released from the body, the available energy can be used to adapt to circumstances in a more positive, constructive way. A byproduct of this is wisdom gained and stronger willpower.

SHOCK

Mental and physical shock scatters Qi, causes a sudden depletion of Heart Qi, and affects the Kidneys. Symptoms may include palpitations, breathlessness, and insomnia.

LOVE

Obsessive love can cause disease when it is misdirected toward a person who hurts you physically or mentally. This type of love affects the Heart and quickens Qi. Symptoms include heart palpitations, a red tip of the tongue, a red face, insomnia, and mental restlessness.

CRAVING

Constant craving of material things or social recognition is common in Western consumer-driven societies. This is largely the result of our endless bombardment with advertising. Craving scatters Qi and affects the Heart and Pericardium. If craving causes Heart Fire, symptoms will include heart palpitations, a red face, thirst, insomnia, agitation, and manic behavior. If there is a tendency to yin deficiency (especially in people who overwork), craving leads to what is called Heart Empty Heat, with palpitations, malar (cheek) flush, dry throat, insomnia, and mental restlessness.

GUILT

The feeling of guilt (which is not the same thing as actually *being* guilty) is also a cause of disease. Some people have a tendency to blame themselves for everything that goes wrong, whether or not the circumstances are actually within their control. They may feel regret for real or imagined deeds (past or present), self-reproach, and a sense of inadequacy or despair.

Guilt is pervasive in Western people, yet it is completely missing from Chinese medicine because guilt does not exist in the Chinese psyche and soul. This is because guilt has its foundations in the Judeo-Christian religions.

It leads to Qi stagnation and may quickly cause blood stasis. Guilt affects all the organs of the body. Symptoms include a purple tongue with a red tip and the "sinking" of Qi (for example, urinary or gynecological problems).

SHAME

Shame is an overwhelming feeling of worthlessness, self-accusation, or being judged all the time. You may feel that you need to hide because you've done something that society frowns upon—for example, something "dirty." This emotion is related to our perception of how we appear to others, not how we feel inside. It's about our place in society—what people see us doing and what they think of it.

As long as we conform to the rules of society or are not seen or found out, we don't feel shame. The danger in shame is that it can produce extreme consequences like hari-kari (suicide) and other forms of self-destruction. Shame is common in both Western and Eastern cultures, but Western societies are more guilt-based and Eastern ones are shame-based. When we feel guilty, we hear an inner voice condemning us, but when we feel shame, we imagine other people condemning us. Shame makes Qi stagnate and possibly sink, creating dampness. Symptoms of shame's impact on the body include organ prolapse, chronic vaginal discharge, chronic excessive menstrual bleeding, and chronic slight urinary incontinence.

DON'T IDENTIFY WITH DISEASE AND PAIN

You now know that emotions that aren't processed properly produce inflammation, which in turn creates the potential for illness. When you combine your constitution, an unhealthy environment, unhealthy food, and a weak genetic disposition, and on top of that pile on a whole lot of suppressed emotion, you're setting yourself up for trouble.

The body works as a whole, and when one part is out of balance, the effects will eventually spread throughout. This is why we need to address the entirety of each person when looking at neck and back pain. There is no one symptom of imbalance that operates in a vacuum; each part of the body is interconnected with the system as a whole. When the organs of the body are not in harmony with one another, disease will result, and every symptom of imbalance is a chance to recognize the need for realignment and respond appropriately. A necessary first step is to avoid identifying with the imbalance and to redirect the mind toward healthier states.

Even something as simple as positive self-talk can have an impact on the level of pain and inflammation in the body. This is because we directly affect our emotions with our thoughts and positive thoughts create a more positive internal environment for our organs. I love mirror talk. It's one of my favorite things to do every morning as I prepare for the day. I do this especially on mornings when I'm not feeling well. I look myself in the eyes and say, "I choose to co-create with God that I love myself and I believe in myself. I choose to co-create that I'm healthy, happy, and vibrant." I also repeat this to myself throughout the day so that I don't focus on any possible symptoms. I don't attach myself to my symptoms. Instead, I focus on what it is that I want. I don't focus on what it is that I *don't* want.

Also, if you're often sick, pay attention, but don't focus on the illness. Don't view the illness as though it identifies you as a person. For example, if you have suffered with chronic back issues or fibromyalgia for many years, remember that you are not your disease. Rephrase the labeling by saying to yourself, "I have a temporary condition called lumbar stenosis that has healed easily and effectively."

Really pay attention to how you talk to yourself and think about your illness, especially if you have a weaker constitution or if you tend to get sick easily.

Instead of identifying with your neck and back pain as a permanent part of your experience, make sure you get enough sleep and adopt the healthy habits I recommend in this chapter. Focus on positive thoughts and actions and soon you'll find yourself on the way to better health.

5

BACK PAIN 101

Now that we have covered the foundations of Chinese medicine and the way imbalance shows up in the body, it's time to get down to business. But before we dive into healing it, let's look at exactly what back pain is.

You can experience back pain whenever there is a malfunction of the spine or any of the many tissues that connect to and influence it—which means there's a lot that can go wrong!

Your spine is composed of a column of bones, called vertebrae, that extend from the the base of the skull to the tip of your tailbone. But your spine doesn't exist in isolation. It's like the trunk of a tree held together by your muscles, tendons, ligaments, and nerves. Each vertebra has a cushioned, shock-absorbing, fluid-filled disc between it and the other vertebrae that assists with movement and ensures that nerves extending from the spine are not compressed.

There are four parts to the spine—cervical (neck), thoracic (middle back), lumbar (lower back), and sacrum/tailbone The spinal column is made up of 33 bones: seven vertebrae in the cervical region, twelve in the thoracic region, five in the lumbar region, five in the sacral region, and four in the tailbone.

The nerves that come out of each vertebra control our extremities, including our hands and feet. Different parts of the spine influence different bodily functions—resting, digesting, sexual function, heartbeat, respiration, our fight-or-flight mechanisms, and the rest of those nonconscious body mechanics that we take for granted, like breathing.

Back pain comes with many related issues, such as drop-leg syndrome; sciatica; lumbar stenosis; herniated, bulging, or ruptured discs; sacroiliac pain; atrophy of the calves; certain types of knee pain; numbness or pain in the toes; plantar fasciitis; and Achilles' heel syndrome. But no matter the cause, Western medicine's standard remedy strategies are not focused on *curing* the conditions, but on *managing* them.

In Chinese medicine, on the other hand, we are always looking for the root cause in order to reverse the condition. Many times the root cause is not in the same place where the dysfunction or pain shows up. For example, the psoas muscle is a main contributor to back pain and its related issues. Western medicine does not look at other areas of the body as potential sites of the root cause of these dysfunctions; it merely focuses on alleviating symptoms at the source of pain—a temporary solution at best.

Two of the most common Western antidotes for back pain are steroidal injections and prescription pain medications. But besides causing other health-related issues such as constipation, diarrhea, impotence, nocturnal emissions, enuresis (involuntary urination), low sex drive, anxiety, and depression, the overprescribing of pain medications is one of the main contributors to the opioid addiction epidemic in our country. Pain management in a more holistic sense would mean reducing pain and increasing someone's ability to move so that their day-to-day life functions were improved through behavioral modifications, physical therapy, massage therapy, and acupuncture.

Symptoms of lower back issues range widely from mild or sharp burning sensations to excruciating pain and debilitation. *Chronic back pain* is defined as pain lasting more than three months. The pain can be *consistent*, meaning you feel it no matter what you're doing, or it can be *intermittent* and have alternating sensations, such as numbness and tingling. Your symptoms may also change locations; you can have sciatic nerve pain for a day or more and then suddenly it changes to pain in the knee or numbness of the big toe. For some, the pain depends on their position. For example, lying on their stomach or on their side makes the pain worse. Walking, standing, or sitting in one position for too long can cause discomfort or pain or there might be a combination of positions that trigger it.

Pain can originate from structural problems (which is most common), or from direct injury to the lower back (for instance, in a car accident). It may also arise from diseases like diabetes or cancer of the spine. The sensations vary: electric shock, numbness, tingling, a sudden jolt, or weakness of the muscles (especially in the legs and calves) all the way down to the feet and toes. There can be tightness or pain in the groin, pain that wraps around the waist, or pain that radiates from the lower lumbar to the buttocks. Sometimes the pain will radiate down the back of the leg or into the thigh and calf. Sometimes the pain has a sudden onset. Something as simple as sneezing or bending over to pick up a tennis shoe can trigger the back, causing intense and debilitating pain.

For some, the pain is gradual and only intensifies as time goes on. This depends on what vertebrae and discs are affected and what nerves are being compressed. Different nerves have different functions and responses to injury. For example, if L4 is compressed, pain will show up quickly in the sciatic nerve, whereas compression in L1 (the tailbone) may take time to manifest in the form of numbness in the buttocks.

Some will notice more back pain during stressful times in their lives or when they're exposed to certain external environmental factors like wind and cold. However, all these symptoms trace their origins back to two root causes: one particularly important muscle and the sympathetic nervous system.

WHAT'S THE PSOAS GOT TO DO WITH IT?

In 1991, I severely injured my back while training in Tae Kwon Do. Doctors were pushing for me to have back surgery. Luckily, my mother, who was a nurse, was working for a doctor by the name of Nancy Bergmann. Dr. Bergmann not only facilitated my healing process but educated me on how the back functions. And, most importantly, she opened my eyes to the importance of having a healthy psoas muscle (see the illustration on the next page). In addition, the therapist working with her at the time was a martial artist, and he is the one that introduced me to Qigong.

I continued to work with Dr. Nancy and devoted myself to a serious daily Qigong regimen. As a result, I was able to fully heal my back—contrary to what some doctors told me was possible. In 1998, Dr. Nancy introduced me to a book called *The Psoas Book* by Liz Koch, first published in 1997. This book became my study guide. Liz not only goes into the function of the psoas but also explores how childhood conditioning, fear, post-traumatic stress disorder (PTSD), and even the menstrual cycle are all controlled by this muscle. She even postulates that the psoas is so important that it has its own soul! I believe Liz is one of the greatest pioneers in educating people about the psoas and its functions.

Fast forward to 2010: my wife Parisa and I met and merged our businesses. We built a beautiful 2,000-square-foot clinical practice space with a Pilates, fitness, and lecture studio in the Willow Glen district of San Jose, California. In this amazing new space, I had the privilege of meeting Liz and hosting a few of her events, bringing it all full circle. I've drawn upon some of her wisdom as well as my own experience with the psoas in the following paragraphs.

The biggest culprit in most back issues is the psoas muscle, also known as the iliopsoas muscle. It is a massive muscle deep inside your abdomen. It's about the width of a fist and is approximately 16 inches long. It indirectly connects the rib cage and trunk with the thighs and legs.

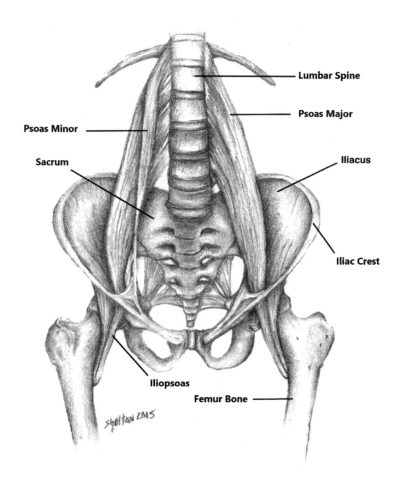

Most people have heard of hip flexors but are unaware of the psoas muscle. Whenever you go to see your doctor, chiropractor, or physical therapist for low back or sciatica issues, the psoas muscle should be number one in conversation. The psoas muscle is basically a hip flexor, and its principal function is to stabilize the spine. The spine doesn't sit straight by itself; it relies on muscles like the psoas.

Since the psoas supports the spine, whenever you have a compressed disc or pinched nerves in the spinal column, it's because the psoas muscle is too tight on one side or the other. Generally both sides are tight, but one side will tend to be tighter than the other. The tighter side compresses vertebrae in the back, causing bulging, ruptured, or deteriorating discs (see sideview illustration of the psoas muscle below). This also causes pain in the sacroiliac joint, aka the SI joint, and compression of the nerves that exit the spinal canal and feed into the trunk of the body and the legs.

The psoas muscle allows your legs to swing easily when you walk, and it plays an essential role in transferring weight from the trunk to the legs and into the feet. This muscle responds to the shift of gravity through the trunk and enables the leg to follow. Therefore, walking isn't initiated in the legs or leg muscles, as you might assume. It's actually initiated by the group of muscles that make up the psoas. If you go to stand up and get a "stuck" feeling in your groin, hear a clicking or popping sensation in the area, or notice that your leg catches as you walk, that's the psoas letting you know that it's tight. These issues are often a precursor to back problems.

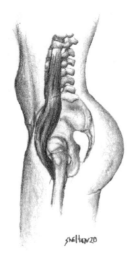

shelton20

The psoas acts as a counterbalance to the abdominal muscles that help maintain a proper front-to-back (anterior–posterior) relationship. So if you notice that you are not standing up straight, it's because of your psoas.

The psoas also connects to the diaphragm and aids in breathing. In addition, it has smaller branches that help to keep your organs in place. Whether your organs sit properly in the visceral cavity is based on how healthy your psoas muscle is.

When your psoas is out of balance and is too tight, it can affect the proper functioning of internal organs. That's because the psoas supports your internal organs and functions like a hydraulic pump. Its movement allows for fluids, such as blood and lymph, to be pushed in and out of cells. If this movement is impaired because the psoas is too tight, it will affect the proper movement of fluids and can have an adverse impact on your internal organ systems. Your psoas runs alongside your entire digestive system and thus can also affect proper movement through your intestines.

The psoas naturally lengthens and shortens as it expands and contracts. When it's in a shortened or continually contracted state from sitting too much or playing sports that require a bent-over posture (like wrestling, bicycling, or certain positions in football), it can cause other structural problems. You may develop a sore back or conditions like scoliosis, lumbar hyperextension, or lumbar stenosis. In addition, your hips may go out of alignment.

As I mentioned earlier, even when the psoas muscles on both sides are tight, one side generally will be tighter, creating another structural issue where one leg is shorter than the other. Unfortunately, some physical therapists and podiatrists remedy this by placing orthotics, or lifts, in the shoe of the shorter leg. These usually aren't necessary and can cause more problems down the line.

Most knee pain, Achilles' heel pain, and plantar fasciitis also stem from a too-tight psoas muscle. It can be the precursor to serious knee problems (like a torn meniscus) and increases the probability of a rollover ankle sprain. Another problem that can arise from a tight psoas is degeneration of the hip and the articular cartilage (see image on the next page), an issue that can lead to hip replacement surgery.

The articular cartilage is the cartilage that's inside the acetabulum (socket) of the hip bone, into which the head of the femur bone fits.

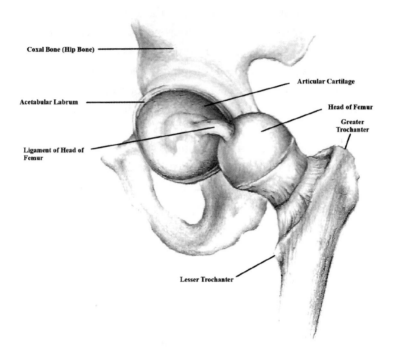

Coxal Bone (Hip Bone)

Articular Cartilage

Acetabular Labrum

Head of Femur

Greater Trochanter

Ligament of Head of Femur

Lesser Trochanter

BACK PAIN'S ROOTS IN EMOTIONAL TRAUMA

It makes sense that physical trauma can cause back pain. We easily accept the idea that activities that keep our psoas contracted for long periods of time, such as excessive sitting, lifting heavy objects inappropriately, and playing certain sports, can spell trouble. But would you be surprised to learn that emotional trauma can also throw your psoas out of balance and cause back pain?

It's true.

Fear is the first big culprit.

As stated earlier, according to Chinese medicine, the negative emotions fear and shock attack the Kidneys and weaken their essence. This is especially relevant because the Kidneys control the lower back.

The Kidneys, in coordination with the Liver and the sympathetic nervous system, are triggered by a fight-or-flight response, directly impacting and causing symptoms in the low back region.

I've personally experienced low back pain and its connection with fear. As a competing martial artist, I would sometimes develop severe low back pain one or two days before a match. Then competition day would come. After the fight was over, my back pain would miraculously disappear!

The Kidneys are also connected to the ears. When a person experiences the fear of falling, the vestibular system is triggered (see two images below). This is the sensory apparatus of the inner ear that helps the body maintain its postural equilibrium, sense of balance, and spatial orientation for the purpose of coordinating movement and balance. The vestibular system must function properly to synchronize head position and eye movement. Thus, when we see clients with tinnitus (ringing in the ears) or Ménière's disease (episodes of vertigo that cause the person to feel as though they are continuously spinning), Western medicine blames the vestibular system in the inner ear. But in reality, the root of the dysfunction lies in the Kidneys.

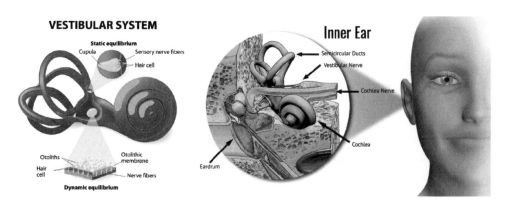

What's scientifically fascinating is that while a fetus is forming in the uterus, the kidneys and ears grow at the same time. Doctors know the baby will have kidney problems if the ears don't properly form in the fetus. For some reason, Western science tends to lose sight of this after the baby is born. As a result, when a person has balance issues, vertigo, or ringing in the ears, instead of remedying the Kidneys, Western medicine tries to treat the inner ear.

At a Christmas party several years ago, I had an in-depth conversation with the head of urology from one of the major hospitals in the San Francisco Bay Area about the connection between the ears and the kidneys. He couldn't get beyond the fact that the major function of the kidneys is secretion and excretion. In Chinese medicine, we understand the function of the internal organs according to science and Western medicine, but we also know these organs have a much greater functionality. I believe that as integrated medicine advances, science will eventually recognize these connections and empower doctors to further help their patients.

The Kidneys also influence the Urinary Bladder. This is why people in flight mode are known to urinate on themselves. In my clinical practice, we sometimes see young adolescents who are suddenly wetting the bed at night and we immediately know there's something going on in the household and that the Kidneys are responsible.

A mother brought her 10-year-old son to see me after several weeks of bedwetting. She said it was a new development and had not been a problem since he was potty-trained as a young boy. I asked the mother if there had been any significant changes in her son's emotional environment. She said, "His father and I are getting a divorce and we are going to have to move, but it is a very amicable separation. He's not seeing any arguing or bickering; we just fell out of love with one another."

I asked the mother to step out of the room so I could talk to her son briefly before I began his therapy session. After I made further inquiry, the young boy explained to me that he was afraid his parents were getting a divorce. He was also afraid of having to move and start over at a new school. This is an example of Kidney Qi descending and affecting the bladder because of fear. It's also a great example of how stress in one's environment can trigger this fight-or-flight mechanism in the body. In this case, it was obvious that the young boy was in flight mode. What was interesting about this situation was that because his mother considered the divorce amicable, she didn't see how big of an impact it was having on her son. After explaining to the mother what I had uncovered and with a few more sessions and specific Qigong practices as well as a rec-ommendation to see a therapist and an Emotional Freedom Technique (EFT) practitioner, the bedwetting stopped.

To sum up: emotional trauma, especially fear, commonly causes back pain. I see it frequently in practice. Fear weakens the Kidneys, and because the Kidneys control the lower back, that fear you're feeling can manifest physically in numerous symptoms related to low-back pain. If you're suffering from any low back pain or related conditions, one of the first things you must do is ask yourself, "What's been going on in my life to create fear?"

The fear response also wreaks havoc on your psoas.

FIGHT-OR-FLIGHT AND THE PSOAS

The psoas is your protection muscle. It is so large and controls so great an area, that if you had to curl up into a ball right away—for example, if you were being attacked or experiencing an earthquake—the psoas would help you do it immediately. That's considered a flight response. To survive, the body will do what it needs to.

The front side of your body is considered the delicate yin side because it encompasses your vital internal organs. The outside, or back of the body, is considered yang and strong. When you curl up into a ball, your yang side is protecting the delicate yin side consisting of the abdomen and chest.

In the clinic, when we see clients who have back issues rooted in the psoas, they walk a little hunched over, sometimes with their shoulders slightly rolled forward. This is because the psoas is in protection mode. It's so tight that it causes the sufferer's posture and structure to round itself. After we loosen the psoas in the groin, the person not only stands up straighter, but their shoulders roll back as well.

My friend and Tae Bo creator, Billy Blanks, told the Denver Nuggets trainer that I helped him grow two inches after I worked on the psoas to help fix his hip pain. The reality is that I didn't help Billy grow two inches. I loosened his psoas, which allowed his posture to straighten, and he stood taller as a result. I said to Billy at the time, "Shoot, if I could help *you* grow two inches, Lord knows I could help myself grow two inches!"

THE ROLE OF STRESS, ANGER, AND RESENTMENT

The next most common emotions that impact proper functioning of the psoas are stress, anger, old anger, and resentment. All these emotions affect the Liver and the Gallbladder.

It works like this: fear (as described in the previous section) is your fight-or-flight/protection response. When you're in this mode, Qi descends from the Kidneys. You can't move and your energy is gone—that's flight.

On the other hand, anger and resentment force energy to rise up, causing your ligaments and tendons to constrict. Imagine holding your fists tightly and being ready for battle. Stress and anger affect your Liver and Gallbladder, which in turn constrict your sinews and tendons. This causes contraction that tightens up on your spine and pulls your psoas tighter. It also activates the sympathetic nervous system that is ready for a fight. To summarize, the flight response is anchored in the Kidneys and the fight response is rooted in the Liver.

Most of the time, back problems are quite simple for me to fix. The only time it's difficult is when someone is holding on to a lot of old anger and resentment. As a matter of fact, the toughest problems I've encountered involved women who held a lot of resentment toward a male figure. I only have difficulty helping clients improve their back pain challenges when those emotions haven't been processed.

A high-profile client reached out to me to help her with severe hip and SI joint problems. In our sessions, we started off with a Q&A. She informed me that her husband had cheated on her with a close friend. On top of this, because of the high position held by this woman, the situation had gone public.

Behind the scenes and unknown to the media, she informed me that her husband would force her to have sex with him even when she didn't want to. She harbored a great deal of anger and resentment toward him and felt that there was no justification for his actions. As a result, her psoas muscle had become extremely tight on both sides, but especially on the right. Her sympathetic nervous system was definitely in fight mode. I tried to work with her, but it was extremely painful for her when trying to get the psoas to release.

I told her that she needed to let go of the resentment because it was causing her severe pain. I assigned her Qigong practices for anger and resentment as well as dietary changes and an herbal regimen to benefit the Liver. Normally, back issues are straightforward and easy to fix. In this case, because of her deep-seated anger and resentment, it was an especially challenging scenario that took quite some time to resolve.

As you'll learn throughout this book, the Liver has many functions according to Chinese medicine. One of those is influencing the sympathetic nervous system and another is controlling the sinews. The sinews, which include the tendons, cartilage, and ligaments, affect our capacity for movement and physical activity. The Liver is responsible for the contraction and relaxation of sinews to ensure free movement of the joints. The sinews' capacity for contraction and relaxation depends on the nourishment provided by the blood in the Liver. When someone has constrained Liver Qi and in particular Liver Blood due to poor diet, unhealthy lifestyle habits, and negative emotions, it will affect the sinews and cause contractions, spasms, and difficulty with flexion and extension. On the other hand, when Liver

Blood is abundant, there is no tightness or stiffness, and the movement of the limbs will flow with ease.

According to Chinese medicine, the Spleen is responsible for the skeletal muscles in the limbs. In his book *The Foundations of Chinese Medicine*, Giovanni Maciocia states that there is an overlap in the pathology and physiology between the Spleen and the Liver as well as the sinews and muscles.

Weakness of the leg muscles is related to the Spleen's function being weakened, whereas contraction (like we see with a tight psoas muscle) is related to the Liver. In clinical practice, one of the ways we remedy the psoas is by working on the Gallbladder acupuncture meridian. When the Liver gets out of balance, it affects the functioning of the Gallbladder. It creates not only organ pathology but acupuncture channel pathology as well.

The sciatic nerve follows the Gallbladder acupuncture meridian down the outside of both legs. When we see clients in the clinic with severe PTSD, I press on these points in the groin along the Gallbladder meridian, and many times the client will have an immediate emotional release. The larger the trauma, the larger the release.

In my clinical practice in San Jose, California, I see military veterans from not only past wars but also the recent war in the Middle East (the one nobody's talking about). These soldiers come in with PTSD. Guess where they store it? In their psoas.

One protocol I use with anyone that comes in with back pain of any type is this: I press on the psoas muscle and the acupuncture points in the groin. Whenever I press on the groin, I get an immediate emotional release. Sometimes it's a violent outburst or uncontrollable sobbing. This emotional release creates a huge healing opportunity. It frees up space in the body, relaxes the nervous system, and they immediately feel lighter. As a result, the sympathetic nervous system gets to relax, the Liver releases, and they heal their own back!

Another example:

A 23-year-old student was referred to me by a friend. She had been diagnosed with lupus two years before and was taking the medications her doctors had prescribed, yet it seemed as if her symptoms were coming back. The doctors were recommending stronger doses of her medications, and she was looking for alternatives because of the negative side effects. She had red, inflamed, itchy blotches on her arms and torso and on the inner canthus (corner) of her left eye. She also had severe pain radiating down her legs, especially on the right side. She was suffering from fatigue as well as pain that would start in her big toe or pinky toe and radiate across all five.

During our first Q&A, the young woman revealed that she didn't like to show when she was angry. She liked everybody to get along and was willing to suck up her own feelings if it meant that someone else could be happy. She came from a very traditional Chinese family where they didn't talk about their emotions and weren't allowed to demonstrate their anger. This case is a fine example of inflammation getting stored in the body when an emotion is not properly expressed. In this case, when she did feel angry or resentful toward something or someone, she would just hold it in. This affected her Liver and sympathetic nervous system. Her repressed emotions showed up as red, inflamed, itchy blotches on her skin. They also tightened her psoas muscle, causing the pain radiating down her legs and into her toes.

I gave her tools to deal with her resentments and anger and explained that anger is not a bad thing. It is there to help us to make a positive change in our world, to fight for the underdog, or to get out of a bad situation. When you suppress anger—or even worse, as in her case, not allow yourself to feel it—it has to show up somewhere inside the body. In this case, it showed up as nerve pain and a skin condition that doctors diagnosed as lupus.

When she left my office after a session, she felt better for several days. I told her that my goal for our work together was to teach her to make a better mind-body connection, meaning that when pain showed up inside her body, she would learn to pause and take a look at what was going on in her outside environment that could be irritating her. I'm glad to say that after several sessions, she started making the mind-body connection. The red blotches on her skin went away and she seldom has tingling, numbness, or pain in her legs, feet, and toes.

THE LINK BETWEEN THE KIDNEYS, THE LIVER, AND THE SYMPATHETIC NERVOUS SYSTEM

What is the sympathetic nervous system and what does it have to do with back pain?

Let's say you're at home eating a black bean burrito when, all of a sudden, the chandelier starts shaking, the ground begins to move, pictures fall off the wall, and you realize you're in the middle of an earthquake. Your heart starts to race, your respiration increases, and you may even begin to sweat. The reason is that you're stressed. Not the kind of stress like "What should I wear to dinner next Friday night with Aunt Susie?" but the stress that you're possibly going to die! Stress is a good thing in this case because it gives us the opportunity to react, get motivated, and get into action (see image below). In these kinds of scenarios, the sympathetic nervous system is responsible for triggering parts of our body, including certain organs, to react so that we can either duck and cover or run from the danger.

NERVOUS SYSTEM

PARASYMPATHETIC

SYMPATHETIC

PARASYMPATHETIC	SYMPATHETIC
PUPIL Constriction	**PUPIL** Dilation
HEART Slows hearbeat	**HEART** Increases hearbeat
CRANIAL — **AIRWAYS** Constricts the bronchial tubules	**AIRWAYS** Dilates the bronchial tubules
CERVICAL — **LIVER** Stimulates bile release	**SWEAT GLAND** Stimulates secretion — CERVICAL
BLOOD VESSELS Dilation	**LIVER** Increases the rate of glycogen-to-glucose conversion
THORACIC — **DIGESTIVE SYSTEM** Stimulates activity	**DIGESTIVE SYSTEM** Decreases activity — THORACIC
	ADRENAL GLANDS Stimulate the production of adrenaline / kidney
LUMBAR — **UTERUS** Relaxes	**UTERUS** Stimulates orgasm — LUMBAR
SACRAL — **URINARY SYSTEM** Increases urinary output	**URINARY SYSTEM** Relaxes bladder — Sympathetic ganglion

The sympathetic nervous system's counterpart is the parasympathetic nervous system. This is mainly responsible for bodily functions that we take for granted, like making reproductive cells, resting, and digesting (as in your black bean burrito). During a high-stress situation like an earthquake, the sympathetic nervous system overrides the parasympathetic nervous system and stops you from digesting the burrito. It transfers the blood from your stomach and intestines to the heart, lungs, and brain while firing up the muscles in your extremities so you can get the heck out of the house. We are so lucky to have a sympathetic nervous system because we would probably die in a short amount of time without it.

Originally, the sympathetic nervous system was there to help us react in dangerous situations: to escape when our house catches fire, to run when we're chased by a bear, or to protect ourselves in an earthquake. Nowadays, this part of the nervous system doesn't know the difference between a survival situation and running late for an appointment or being behind in paying the bills or any of the other numerous external stresses that society places upon us.

Jose, a star high school basketball player, was on course to receive a full athletic scholarship to a prestigious university. One night during a championship game, he performed a layup to try to score a point. While in the air, he was hit by another player on the opposite team. Jose fell to the floor. The wind was knocked out of him, but after sitting for a few minutes he was able to go back in and finish the game.

Two days later, he tried to get out of bed but had difficulty walking and even moving. Doctors performed an MRI and ran X-rays, diagnosing him with lumbar stenosis. Their treatment strategy was bed rest and cortisone spinal injections. The injections seemed to work at first, but over time their effectiveness ceased. Doctors were now telling him that he needed spinal surgery and would never play basketball again.

Jose's mom heard about me from Hollywood physique expert Eric the Trainer, and she flew me out to Chicago to help her son. I had Jose do the psoas stretch, and I pressed on certain acupuncture points in the groin as well as on the SI joint. With that remedy, I had Jose running and jumping in 15 minutes! After that successful session, his mom would occasionally fly us out to Illinois to help people in their community, including other players on Jose's basketball team. On the way home to California after one such trip, I wondered, Why are these young kids being diagnosed with back issues that, in the past, would only have affected higher-risk older people?

That's when I made the connection to the sympathetic nervous system. And what hit me like a ton of bricks was that these days, our sympathetic nervous systems are being activated all the time. We are constantly under stress that affects the Liver and allows for these conditions to show up in otherwise young, healthy, active adults. Nowadays, our sympathetic nervous systems are being triggered nonstop by the pressures of everyday life. Screen time, social media, and incessant bombardment with other media messages only worsen that stress.

In the case of these young basketball players, they faced the stressors of getting accepted into the university of their choice, keeping their grades up, and outperforming their teammates—not to mention whatever stress was going on in their personal lives and homes.

As another example, a client of mine was angry about the political news and discussions he saw regularly on Facebook. I advised him to disconnect immediately. Two weeks later, his back was doing much better. So think about the stresses in your life. Your trigger may not be social media; it could be other people in your environment, pollution, or even eating too many genetically modified and processed foods.

It's important to understand what's going on chemically inside your body when you're continually under stress. It's critical that you realize how stress will not only affect your back but cause many other diseases.

According to Chinese medicine, one of the many functions of the Liver is its role in the nervous system. When your sympathetic nervous system is constantly overactive and in a state of heightened arousal or agitation, it's considered to be in a yang state. If the parasympathetic nervous system was underactive or in the *off* position, this would be considered yin; you'd be paralyzed or in a frozen state.

In short, from a Chinese medicine point of view, there are two organs that have influence on the sympathetic nervous system: the Liver and the Kidneys. The myriad of ways neck and back pain show up can be traced back to these main organs, and addressing the causes of their imbalance will allow the body to realign naturally, without the need for medication or surgery.

Now that you've got the background, let's answer the question that's burning in your mind: "What the heck do I do about it?"

6

BACK PAIN AND YOUR FIVE ELEMENT TYPE

If you took the Five Element Questionnaire and your result was that you're predominantly a Wood type or that your weakest element is Wood, you may be more prone to low and mid-back issues. If you haven't taken the quiz yet, scan the QR code below or head over to http://chrissheltonseasyguide.com.

When taking the quiz, you will learn about the Five Element personalities: Fire, Earth, Metal, Water, and Wood. When Wood types are out of balance, their go-to emotions are anger, resentment, frustration, old anger, and control (as in trying to be controlling).

I understand this because when I was a child, my environment was always unsettled. When I got older, I thought that if I controlled all situations and events, I could control the outcomes. When you're behaving in a controlling way, you tend to be rigid and hold on to things too tightly. And if you hold onto situations too tightly, your muscles will tighten in the low and middle back.

Also, holding on to anger or repressed resentment creates heat in the Liver. Furthermore, if blood and Qi get stuck in the Liver, this will cause it to expand. You may then notice pain in the rib cage or referred pain in the middle back, also known as a "side stitch." (Referred pain is when you have a dysfunction or injury in one area of the body but feel the pain somewhere else.)

The key is to learn how to let go and allow space in all situations. To help create space, you can incorporate Tai Chi and Qigong into your daily routine or you can use a mantra. Look at yourself in the mirror and say, "I have complete acceptance of all situations." This will help if you're a person who likes to be in control. If you want to use a mantra to eliminate anger and resentment, recite what you want to create instead to bring more of *that* into your life—for example, "I choose to co-create with God that I am loving and compassionate toward myself and all people."

Even though back pain is more frequent among Wood-predominant or Wood-deficient types, any of the Five Element types can suffer from low or mid-back pain. The main issue is when the Liver isn't able to do its job of ensuring the smooth flow of blood and Qi. When there is stagnation or deficiency of Qi, blood, or both, it will affect the Liver's influence on the tendons, ligaments, and sinews as well as on the sympathetic nervous system. It will also cause a deficiency of the Gallbladder and, in particular, the Gallbladder acupuncture meridian, which flows through the groin to the buttocks and follows the sciatic nerve down to the pinky toe. You may develop pain anywhere along that meridian.

THE WOOD ARCHETYPE

You can often tell by looking at someone if they are a Wood type. The major physical signs of Wood types are sinewy tendons and a hard body. Their strength is in their ligaments, tendons, and sinews. They may also have fairly broad shoulders. They tend to look like either tall, slender trees or short, compact bushes.

Their facial shape is rectangular or an inverted trapezoid, and they usually have a protruding brow bone and thick eyebrows (unless they tweeze). The sharper the angles and features on a face (especially around the jawline, cheekbone, brow bone, and eyebrows), the more likely the person is to really enjoy being in charge—and Wood types enjoy being in charge and having control over situations. Add a large nose to this type of face, and you have a very powerful and controlling person.

Wood people constantly need to be *doing* something. They enjoy arguments and discussions, feel compelled to exercise, and love to work hard. These types are seen as aggressive and assertive and often hold their fists clenched. Wood people are action-oriented and quick to take offense. But their rashness can sometimes lead to accidents. If you're a Wood type, pay attention to how you deal with anger and resentment.

Wood types are also prone to injuries of overuse, such as strained, pulled, or torn muscles and tendons. In severe cases of Wood element overuse, conditions like Parkinson's may arise, where movement and coordination are compromised and ultimately impeded.

Wood deficiency, on the other hand, leads to various conditions of exhaustion, including chronic fatigue. Wood people have very strong Livers and enjoy processing toxins, whether emotional (caused by anger) or chemical (as in drugs and alcohol). However, with Wood deficiency, their Livers can become toxified, creating Wood stagnation—especially when they do not release old anger and resentments. This leads to sensitivities to environmental toxins or problems like nausea and headaches. Wood-deficient people are also prone to addiction.

Wood types resist aging. They fight the weakening of their bodies and try to maintain previous levels of activity, both physically and emotionally. It is important for them to practice flexibility instead of rigidity.

On the positive side, the Wood element represents growth, creativity, and awakening. Its nature is expansive and provides a sense of direction for achieving goals. The Wood type is very sociable, can resolve problems easily, and turns ideas into profits. They are hard workers, have good verbal skills, and are extroverts who enjoy completing tasks on their to-do lists.

Wood types tend to have strong tempers and get frustrated easily, especially when others don't come through with their obligations. On the positive side, this tendency to express themselves through their tempers can manifest as hard work, athleticism, and a fighting spirit. They may tend to spread themselves too thin and may also have difficulty expressing their innermost feelings, which can lead to Liver Blood stagnation and depression. Yet Wood folks can handle tremendous amounts of pressure and strict deadlines.

Although anger can be toxic, it is dangerous to Wood people only when used too much or too little. Wood people feel alive when they're in action, and their anger is a wonderfully motivating force for them.

Wood types tend to have stronger Liver Qi than other typologies. The Liver is an amazing organ. It likes processing toxins and then regenerating. It enjoys dealing with poisonous substances and clearing them from the body—unless, of course, it has too many to deal with. At that point, disease may start to show up.

Because the Liver also handles environmental toxins, people with strong Liver Qi can process drugs and alcohol better than others. They tolerate herbal medicines well too, which are part of the Wood family in nature but are also mildly toxic. In fact, most people with strong Liver Qi are capable of tolerating substance abuse (of course this does not mean they *will* abuse substances). People with limited Liver Qi would suffer from alcohol poisoning long before they became alcoholics.

The strength of the Wood element is the ability to be active, both physically and emotionally. Features associated with the Liver show an orientation toward action, temper, the desire for altered states, determination, and issues with authority. The vital feature of the Wood element is the eyebrows, and this is the feature that most closely reflects how well the Liver is functioning. The expression of the Wood element can be seen as fighting for the underdog, creating positive change in the world or one's environment, and doing something creative, such as building things or other forms of artistic self-expression.

THE LIVER AND THE WOOD ELEMENT

The Liver is in the upper right part of the abdomen and works with the Gallbladder. The associated acupuncture channels are on the right and left sides of the body, starting on the inner corners of both big toenails and entering the Liver along the ribs, underneath the nipples.

The main functions of the Liver are to smooth and regulate the flow of vital energy and blood, to store and regulate blood, and to nurture the tendons, nails, and eyes. The Wood element controls the sense of sight and opens into the eyes. If Liver Blood is stagnant, eating foods with a sour taste helps.

Liver Qi is most abundant during the hours of 11:00 p.m. to 3:00 a.m. (the Gallbladder from 11:00 p.m. to 1:00 a.m. and the Liver from 1:00 a.m. to 3:00 a.m.). It's during this time that the blood returns to the Liver to be cleansed.

The positive virtues of Wood types are kindness and creativity. Disease shows up when anger, frustration, hate, old anger, and resentments (toward oneself, others, or both) are not processed properly. Individuals with an excess or deficiency of the Wood element may be prone to sudden outbursts of anger and problems with the nerves, eyes, digestion, tendons, and depression.

But remember that anger is not always bad or negative. All our emotions, including anger, let us know what is going on in our external and internal environments. Anger acts as a positive force when it allows you to express creativity, get out of a bad situation, or fight for the underdog.

THE LIVER'S FUNCTIONS

As discussed, the Liver's main job is smoothing and regulating the flow of vital energy and blood.

The Liver is often compared to Wood in classical Chinese medicine (CCM) because both trees and the Liver tend to "spread out freely." As trees spread their branches, the Liver's function is to spread Qi throughout the body. There are three ways the Liver accomplishes this: regulating mind and mood, promoting digestion and absorption, and keeping Qi and blood moving normally.

According to Chinese medicine, the Heart and the Liver control our mental activities. When the Liver is functioning well, it helps regulate the flow of vital energy and blood, which contributes to psychological health and results in happiness, relaxation, and sensitivity.

When the Liver is not functioning well, the results are anxiety, sighing, sadness, and belching. When the Liver is in terrible health, one may have dizziness, headaches, insomnia, and nightmares.

The Liver's function of regulating the flow of energy throughout the body affects the flow of Qi. If the Liver is not functioning well, the flow of Qi is adversely affected, and this may result in pain in the chest or lower abdomen. And because Qi directly affects blood circulation, when the Liver does not function optimally, the distribution of blood and Qi becomes obstructed.

The Liver aids the Spleen in distributing nutrients and water throughout the body and therefore contributes to proper digestion. An unhealthy Liver can affect the Spleen negatively, resulting in reduced appetite, belching, vomiting, and diarrhea.

Besides being at the root of major back issues, Liver dysfunction can cause the following conditions (and others not mentioned here):

- Pains in the chest and lower abdomen
- Flowery vision (when everything in the periphery is like moving waves)
- Blurred vision
- Numbness of the extremities
- Dry nails
- Unsettled sleep
- Menstrual irregularities, clotting, pain, PMS
- Amenorrhea or menorrhagia
- Hypochondriac pain
- Ringing in the ears
- Chemical sensitivities
- Tumors
- Temporomandibular joint (TMJ) problems
- Distension of the abdomen
- Muscular sclerosis

- Rheumatoid arthritis
- Hives and skin lesions
- Rash
- Facial neuralgia
- Sexual dysfunctions
- Eye or facial tremors
- Convulsions
- Uneven energy throughout the day
- Migraine headaches
- Constipation
- Nausea
- Dizziness
- Crohn's disease
- Colitis
- Allergies
- Fibromyalgia
- Bell's palsy
- Tourette's syndrome
- Stroke and aneurysm

That's not all; Liver imbalances can affect your emotions as well as your physical health.

EMOTIONAL SIGNS OF LIVER IMBALANCE

If your Liver is out of balance, here are some things you may notice:

- Feeling depressed
- Experiencing sudden outbursts of anger
- Feeling overwhelming rage and anger
- Being unable to handle stressful situations
- Having suicidal thoughts
- Experiencing disturbed sleep
- Unable to make plans and follow through

Does that seem like a lot to deal with? It is! The following sections will help you understand why these symptoms show up and what you can do about them.

As you read through this book, remember that by keeping the Liver in balance, we can help the body heal the chronic pain and inflammation of neck and back pain. We can identify and remedy the underlying, causal elements of these imbalances instead of simply masking their symptoms.

THE LIVER AND THE ETHEREAL SOUL

It's important to remember that when we talk about the Liver (with a capital L), we're talking about more than the physical organ itself. We're talking about the spiritual aspects associated with the organ according to Chinese medicine.

Don't worry, I'll explain.

In Chinese medicine, each of the five significant organs has its own "soul," and each of these souls has a clinical function inside the body. When people experience certain diseases or symptoms, having an understanding of the souls not only gives them an excellent diagnostic tool but also helps them find the root of the issue more quickly.

The Liver houses what is known as the Ethereal Soul. The concept of the Ethereal Soul is closely linked to the ancient Chinese belief in spirits and demons. According to these beliefs, spirits and demons are spirit-like creatures that preserve a physical appearance and wander in the world of spirits. Some are good, and some are evil. Prior to the Warring States period (475–221 BC), such spirits were considered the leading cause of disease. Since then, belief in natural causes of disease (such as the weather and the seasons) has replaced this belief, although it has never really disappeared, even to this day.

The Ethereal Soul is yang in nature, and at death, it survives the body to flow back into a world of subtle, nonmaterial energies, or Heaven. In contrast, the Corporeal Soul, housed in the Lungs, is considered yin and returns to Earth at the time of death. The Corporeal Soul is responsible for the physical manifestations in one's life. The main difference between the Corporeal and Ethereal souls is that at the time of death the Ethereal Soul returns to Heaven and the Corporeal Soul returns to Earth.

It's said that a ghost manifests when someone has too strong an attachment to something on the physical plane. Whether it's an attachment to a loved one, money, a house, or another possession, the Corporeal Soul becomes too heavy to ascend.

The Ethereal Soul is said to influence our ability to plan and find a sense of direction in life. A lack of direction and mental confusion can be compared to the wandering of the Ethereal Soul alone in space and time. Thus, if the Liver (in particular, Liver Blood) is flourishing, the Ethereal Soul is firmly rooted and can help us plan our life with wisdom and vision. If Liver Blood is weak, the Ethereal Soul is not rooted and cannot give us a sense of direction in life. If Liver Blood or Liver yin is very weak, the Ethereal Soul may even leave the body temporarily at night, during sleep or just before we go to sleep. Those who suffer from severe deficiency of Liver yin may feel as if they are floating away a few moments before falling asleep. Or they may be almost asleep and suddenly feel their whole body jerk awake. That is said to be the soul returning to the body. Both sensations are believed to be due to the Ethereal Soul not being rooted because of a weakness in the Liver.

The Ethereal Soul is also the source of life dreams, vision, aims, projects, inspiration, creativity, and ideas. It is described as "the coming and going of the Mind" (or Shen). This means that it gives the Mind the necessary other dimensions of life mentioned above: dreams, vision, aims, etc. Without these, the Mind would be sterile and one might suffer from depression.

On the other hand, the Mind needs to restrain the coming and going of the Ethereal Soul somewhat to keep it in check. In essence, the Mind needs to integrate all the ideas spurting forth from the Ethereal Soul into our psyche in an orderly fashion. The Ethereal Soul is like an ocean of ideas, dreams, projects, and inspirations, and the Mind can cope with only one at a time. If the Ethereal Soul brings forth too much material from its ocean without enough control and integration by the Mind, a person's behavior can become somewhat chaotic and, in extreme cases, manic.

When the Ethereal Soul is in balance, it's connected to what is referred to as the objective observer, or Higher Knowing. This Higher Knowing is the voice of intuition or, as some put it, communicating with God. The more you pay attention and act on the direction given by this objective observer, the more it becomes an all-encompassing part of your being. Thus, because the Liver houses this soul, having a healthy Liver also helps promote the evolution of the Ethereal Soul in connection with our higher states of consciousness.

For example, let's say you're going for a walk around the park and your inner voice says, "Bring your checkbook." You think to yourself, "That's ridiculous, I'm just going for a walk around the park." Then, halfway around the park, you run across one of the neighbors' children selling cookies for a fundraiser. Suddenly you're glad you listened to your intuition. The less attention you pay to this internal voice, the less it becomes an all-encompassing part of your being. The more you pay attention to it, the more integrated it becomes in your day-to-day life.

Next up: how to bring your Liver back into balance.

WHAT TO AVOID FOR LIVER HEALTH

Addressing Liver health is essential to healing your neck and back pain, and if you've been experiencing any of the physical or emotional symptoms of a Liver that's out of balance, you can start by incorporating these healthy habits. Don't worry if you can't do everything all at once. It may take time, but start where you feel most comfortable and add new habits once you've established the first ones. You'll notice the difference. I promise!

- Avoid greasy, fatty, and fried foods; excessive alcohol; and sugar. Even ice-cold drinks can make symptoms worse. If you crave those foods, it is a further sign of imbalance.

- Avoid drinking coffee, black tea, and caffeinated sodas.

- Cut out thick, creamy, or cheesy sauces; hot spices; chilies; and large, rich meals. All of these will cause energy to get stuck in the Liver.

- Don't let stress override your system and keep you awake at night. Let go of resentments and anger because they do not serve you. They only accumulate in your system and create the potential for disease.

- Avoid windy conditions. This includes artificial wind from air conditioners in your home or car. Avoid falling asleep with the fan blowing directly on you or sleeping close to an open window where a draft can blow on you.

- Avoid doing things that prevent you from getting a restful night's sleep. If possible, avoid being up after 11:00 p.m. and especially between the hours of 1:00 and 3:00 a.m. when most blood is returned to the Liver for cleansing.

- Avoid watching violent or horror movies, especially before bed.

- Try to avoid being around angry people and having intense, heated conversations. Also, try to avoid spending a lot of time in situations where you feel stuck or trapped.

- Don't repress your emotions. Instead, express what you're feeling.

- Don't let your work life prevent you from exercising or having a creative outlet.

That's the wrap on your Liver for any of the Five Element types.

No matter what your type, if your quiz showed that your Wood element is out of balance, add these strategies as well.

BALANCING YOUR WOOD ELEMENT

If your Wood element is either too prominent or deficient, there are things you can do.

1. FENG SHUI BASIC REMEDIES

Note that there are different schools of feng shui. The remedies I recommend are from the Five Element school.

The color green reflects the Wood element and helps overcome a deficient Wood state. To add more green to your environment, place live plants around your house. You can also add green to your bedspread, curtains, rugs, or pictures or wear more green clothing and jewelry. Also helpful is incorporating furniture made of wood into your home, as well as things that are reminiscent of trees, such as columns or towers, or even a rectangular green candle.

2. GET OUTSIDE

Spending time in forests and surrounding yourself with plants or other forms of vegetation benefits deficient Wood types. No matter where you live, you can find creative ways to adapt. Add some houseplants to your home if you have a small urban apartment or take a drive on the weekends to enjoy a hike in nature.

3. LOWER YOUR STRESS LEVEL

Exercise, and again, make it a point to get outdoors. Practices like Tai Chi, yoga, and Qigong are excellent ways to destress. You can also take a brisk walk or go biking, swimming, jogging, or dancing. Martial arts are highly recommended. Singing and chanting do wonders to lower your stress levels.

4. RECOMMENDED FOODS

See the "What to Avoid for Liver Health" section above for dietary recommendations.

In addition, if you notice that you suffer from anger-related issues, adding sour foods such as lemon, lime, and vinegar to your diet will be very beneficial, if done in moderation.

5. OTHER HELPFUL ACTIVITIES

Be creative! You can write, paint, craft, sculpt, play music, dance, sing, or build something.

Practice sharing your feelings with others. Start small if you're not comfortable doing this.

Learn to pause and take moments throughout your day for a deep breath. Post reminders or set alarms for yourself if you need to.

Journal at night before going to bed and start your morning by listing ten things that you're grateful for. Even a few minutes of journaling each day is beneficial.

Make sure to have good air circulation and sunlight, especially in your bedroom, if possible. Surround yourself with fresh green plants and flowers.

As long as the ground is not cold and wet, walking barefoot outside and feeling a connection to the earth helps cleanse the Liver.

Most of all, don't believe that you have to accept as permanent any of the symptoms or conditions that you're experiencing. Trust the steps I've laid out for you and start embracing better health today.

Wood types aren't the only ones prone to back pain. Let's look at Water types next.

BACK PAIN AND NATURE'S WATER TYPES

Water types also tend to experience back pain more commonly than others. In this section, you'll learn why and what to do about it.

THE WATER ARCHETYPE

If you took the Five Element Questionnaire and came out predominantly as a Water type, you're known as the Sage, or the Survivor. When you are in your strength or in a flow state, you tend to be trusting, energetic, willful, and ambitious and you're able to transform a crisis into an opportunity. You tend to go with the flow. You're confident and have a strong sense of self.

The major physical signs of Water types are a strong back, big bones, and wide hips—Water people carry weight in their hips and thighs. They often look multiethnic, which gives them an exotic, mysterious, or secretive persona. They are prone to shadows around the eyes and have round cheeks and a round face.

Water people are quiet and observant. They are good listeners and give good advice because they have innate wisdom. They appear to be easygoing but when working are very persistent. Water types require a lot of sleep, rest, meditation, or time to just "be." They are strong people, both physically and emotionally. They handle catastrophes and emergencies calmly and tend to have an exaggerated sex drive.

If you're a Water type, you may notice that you like to wear the colors blue and black and you enjoy being around water. The Water element relates to the strength of the Kidneys. In Chinese face reading, the Water element can be seen in the size of the ears and the philtrum, the size of the chin, the under-eye area, and the earlobes.

If your quiz results show that you are deficient in the Water element, you need to beware of being too willful or stubborn. Your main health problems come from the frozen state of Water, which encourages overgrowth of tumors or high blood pressure due to not allowing your emotions to flow. Another potential problem is stagnant Water, where the Water element is not accessible or is unusable. This affects your thinking and is implicated in mental illness and depression. You may notice that you have adrenal burnout; are distrusting, cautious, suspicious, or fearful, or have a false sense of bravado.

Deficient Water occurs when your lifestyle is too active and your Water energy is not replenished. Burning the candle at both ends, poor lifestyle habits, and having too many orgasms all steal your essence. This causes aging and degeneration of the body as well as problems with infertility and impotence.

Water deficiency can be seen in the following conditions: loss of bone density and teeth, deafness, thinning hair, osteoarthritis, and bladder weakness. Genetic defects are also considered a primary form of Water deficiency. However, strong Water energy usually leads to longevity. You strengthen your Water element when you live life wisely and conserve your energy rather than spending it.

THE KIDNEYS' FUNCTIONS

Remember, in addition to the Liver, the Kidneys play a main role in the formation of neck and back pain. Therefore, by understanding more about their functions and how to keep them in balance, greater overall health can be restored, freeing up your body and allowing for the resolution of chronic pain and inflammation. Furthermore, as we become more educated about the ways Kidney imbalance shows up in the body, we can take early steps to restore harmony and prevent further symptoms from developing.

The Kidneys are located on either side of the spinal column. Their main functions are storing the essence of life, regulating water metabolism, and controlling and promoting respiration. Because of this, the Kidneys are related to the Water element.

The Kidneys connect with the Urinary Bladder and the reproductive system (including the testes and ovaries) as well as the endocrine system (including the adrenals, hypothalamus, thyroid, pituitary gland, pineal gland, and thymus). The Kidneys rule the bones, bone marrow, and teeth. Your teeth are considered a surplus of bones.

The Kidneys also relate to the ears. Remember that as a fetus is forming, the kidneys and ears grow at the same time. If you ever see statues or pictures of Buddha, you will notice that his ears are so large that they rest on his shoulders; this represents the strength of his vitality and longevity. His big belly represents the abundance of Qi that is stored in his Kidneys and lower Tan Tien.

The ancient Taoists used to say that if the ears and Kidneys are harmonized, the ear can hear all five tones. The five tones are Gong (do), Shang (re), Jue (mi), Zhi (so), and Yu (la) and can be used to analyze and remedy mind-body illness. The five tones are connected to the internal organs as follows: shouting for the Liver, laughing for the Heart, singing for the Spleen, weeping for the Lungs, and groaning for the Kidneys. By listening to someone's tone of voice, we can sometimes tell what Five Element typology he or she is and/ or what organ is out of balance.

The strength of your Kidney essence also shows up in the moistness and vitality of the hair on your head. Hair depends on blood for nourishment, which is why the hair on your head is referred to as a surplus of blood. The surplus of blood is also an extension of the Kidneys, and healthy, luxurious hair is a sign that your Kidney essence is strong. Thus, if you have dry or withered hair, are balding, are experiencing premature graying, or are losing hair prematurely, it is due weakness of the blood and essence of the Kidneys.

The Kidneys rule what the Chinese call the "grasping" of Qi, and the Lungs govern respiration. Normal breathing requires assistance from the Kidneys. The Kidneys enable the natural air to penetrate deeply, completing the inhalation process mentioned above as the "grasping" of Qi.

When a client comes in complaining of shortness of breath and states that they have difficulty inhaling, I know the Kidneys are at the root of the dysfunction, since they work along with the Lungs and aid in inhalation. When the Kidneys aren't functioning well, you will exhale more than you inhale, which can result in dyspnea (labored respiration) and even panting.

The Kidney system is most abundant with Qi during the hours of 3:00 p.m. to 7:00 p.m. (Bladder 3:00–5:00 p.m., Kidneys 5:00–7:00 p.m.).

Here is the easiest way to find your kidneys: Imagine sticking a dowel through your belly and directly out your back. That imaginary dowel will land right between the left and right kidneys. The adrenal glands rest on top of the Kidneys and are the most sensitive of all yin organs. They are almost always deficient and almost never in excess. The only exception occurs in some cases where the Urinary Bladder is in excess and out of balance, creating an excess condition inside the Kidneys.

If you crave salty foods and tend to wear blue or black frequently, there is a possibility that you are weak in the Water element. Kidney weakness is common among Americans and shows up as physical weakness and a lack of energy. If you find that you are running to Starbucks at three to five o'clock in the afternoon to get that pick-me-up, signs point to a Kidney weakness. If you're deficient in another element type and have any of the above symptoms, it still means the Kidneys are weak and could be contributing to the condition.

Because the kidneys secrete and excrete, they maintain the balance of fluid in the body. Fluid in the body is responsible for transporting nutrients to organs and tissues, and it aids in getting rid of waste. The kidneys play an important role in both functions, either by releasing water or retaining needed water. When they are functioning well, urination is normal. When in dysfunction, they can release too much, causing conditions like frequent urination. When the kidneys do not release enough, it can lead to edema and swelling of the extremities.

In Chinese medicine, the Kidney system does much more than just filter water. It also stores the essence of life (sperm and eggs) while controlling the bones, bone marrow, and brain (called the sea of marrow). This influences growth, maintenance, and reproduction; produces blood; and opens to, or controls, the ears. The adrenals are included within the Kidney system; thus adrenal exhaustion is Kidney exhaustion. Weakness of the Kidneys often manifests as problems in the back, knees, ears, or reproductive functions. The Kidneys greatly influence health and longevity.

Kidney function (and resulting problems) can be divided into Kidney yang and Kidney yin.

THE KIDNEYS AND THE ROOT OF YIN AND YANG

This essence contained in the Kidneys is connected to life itself. It is the source of life and gives life its specific character. It's the basis for growth and development. It's also the foundation of yin and yang. The entire body and all the organs need the balance of yin and yang in order to thrive. For a visual of yin and yang, please refer to page 14.

The yin aspect of the Kidneys, housed in the left Kidney, is the storing of water. Kidney yin is the foundation for all cooling and lubricating substances inside the body. It is the basis for sweat, blood, bodily fluids, spinal fluids, digestive fluids, synovial fluids, and others. See image below.

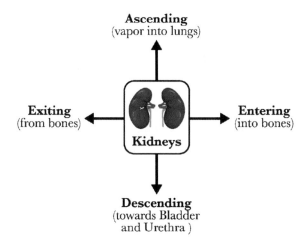

This can be confusing. We all know blood is warm, but because of its nourishing and lubricating function, it's considered yin. As an analogy, consider the radiator fluid in your car. Even though radiator fluid gets hot, it circulates throughout the engine and transmission to help cool it and keep it from overheating. Without radiator fluid, the engine block would crack due to the excessive heat and friction generated by the moving parts.

The yang aspect, which is stored in the right Kidney, is referred to as the Life Gate of Fire and is the heat, or motive force, for transformation in the body. For example, it takes heat to move blood to the extremities, cause your heart to beat, and enable your stomach to digest food.

Since the Kidneys are the root of yin and yang for the entire body, if yin and/or yang is deficient in the Kidneys, chances are that it will be deficient in other organs as well. All Kidney patterns are normally considered deficient patterns unless we are talking about the Urinary Bladder. In that case, there can be a combined deficient/excessive type. Imbalances of Kidney yin and yang are at the root of both the pathology and physiology of dysfunction. Since Kidney yin is responsible for the essence and fluids in the body and Kidney yang for the motive force of transformation in the body, when you have a weakness in one, at some level you have a weakness in the other.

The Kidneys are also at the root of our pre-Heaven essence and are always affected in any chronic disease. When there is not enough essence of life for the five major organs and corresponding bowels, the Kidneys will supply it. Thus, when any of the five major organs and corresponding bowels are not functioning correctly, the Kidneys need to be nourished and strengthened in order to harmonize the imbalance in whatever organs or organ systems are affected.

If you suffer from night sweats, there is a weakness of Kidney yin. That's because sweat is yin and the body is sweating because it feels too hot. The body would not do this if there was a proper balance of yin. The problem is that when the body tries to rectify this imbalance through sweating, it continues to sweat and depletes even more yin. When Kidney yang is deficient or when there's not enough heat, it will show up as cold extremities, a sensation of being cold, a white sallow complexion, and certain conditions such as Raynaud's disease and edema.

PHYSICAL SIGNS OF KIDNEY IMBALANCES

If you notice any of these physical conditions, it may mean that your Kidneys are weak and out of balance. Therefore, it is of particular importance that we pay attention to these when experiencing chronic neck and back pain. Recognizing these symptoms early is crucial in establishing lasting balance.

- Weak wilting of the legs and pain or stiffness in the lower lumbar region

- Low back pain

- Diminished cerebral functions in adults and the elderly

- Dizziness

- Poor vision
- Weak bones
- Diminished bone density
- Tremors
- Ringing in the ears
- Loss of coordination
- Stunted growth
- Lack of energy
- Poor memory
- Delayed closure of the fontanels in infancy
- Lack of sex drive

- Infertility
- Shortness of breath
- Hearing loss
- Enuresis (involuntary urination)
- Frequent urination
- Certain types of arthritis
- Bone degeneration
- Premature hair loss and/ or graying
- Involuntary loss of semen

EMOTIONAL SIGNS OF KIDNEY IMBALANCES

If your Water element is weak or unbalanced, it can show up as any of the following:

- Feeling fearful or apprehensive
- Lack of motivation to get out of bed or even to live
- Inability to confront issues
- Inertia

- Lack of motivation and drive
- Lack of willpower
- Brain fog
- Depersonalization disorder
- Anxiety disorder

- Angry outbursts

- Obsession with sex and pornography

- Obsession with masturbation

- Inability to reach orgasm

- Avoidance of intimacy

- No sex drive

STORING OUR LIFE ESSENCE AND CONSTITUTION

The Kidneys store the essence of life and rule our birth and development.

There are two ways in which the Kidneys store our essence. The first is our pre-Heaven Qi. That's our congenital essence of life, meaning it comes from our parents and ancestors. It is further developed at birth and strengthened through proper nutrition. It can be transformed into Qi and is called "the Qi of the Kidney." This Qi of the Kidney contributes to growth, development, and replacement in the body; for example, the growth, development, and replacement of teeth. The body grows as this Qi gets richer and richer. By the time one reaches puberty, Kidney Qi is at its highest. It contributes to the development of sperm in boys and eggs and menstruation in girls. When the body is old, Qi of the Kidney becomes weaker, making reproductive capabilities weaker in turn.

The hereditary constitution of a child is based on the pre-Heaven Qi of his or her parents. (See page 43 for the image of what makes up our hereditary constitution.) Therefore, if the parents' essence is weak at the time of conception or if they conceive late in life, the child's essence will also be weak. This may cause a child to have poor bone development, some mental retardation, loose teeth, frequent urination, bedwetting, and/or thin hair.

The second type of life essence is known as the "acquired" essence of life. This is our post-Heaven Qi. It is derived from food. Our Spleen and Stomach transform the food we eat into acquired essence. That's why it's so important to eat healthy foods, especially those that are good for your constitutional typology. It helps maintain Kidney Qi while slowing the aging process and the degeneration of our tissues.

THE KIDNEYS AND WILLPOWER

Remember, each of the five major organs is said to house a soul. The term *soul* as used here represents the immaterial, emotional, and intellectual aspects of a human being and shows up in one's actions, such as persevering through challenges. The Kidneys house the soul that manifests as our willpower.

There are two aspects of willpower, the yang and the yin. The yang aspect of willpower in the Kidneys inspires you to want to make decisive efforts and fundamental commitments that allow you to take responsibility for your life.

The yin aspect of willpower is recognizing what you desire and believe about how life unfolds. It is based on your intentions and doesn't require much work. The yin aspect of willpower is about the direction we move toward what can only be seen or noticed when we look back and realize how much we have developed over time. It is about our fate, destiny, the unknown, and death.

Contained within willpower are the positive virtues of wisdom and gentleness. Since our Kidneys are our battery of life, what we've learned from the suffering in our lives develops wisdom and teaches us how to have more gentleness and compassion concerning a situation, person, or event. The Taoists say that a sage can't become a sage without suffering. When we let go of the perceived negative aspect of our suffering (pain) and allow learning or wisdom to blossom, we truly develop as spiritual beings and become more in harmony with God.

The Kidneys connect to the ears and the yin urogenital orifice—the urethra and penis in men, the urethra and vagina in women, and the anus. Having a strong sense of hearing and a urinary bladder that is easily able to eliminate its contents are signs of well-functioning Kidneys. Weak Kidneys can result in poor urinary bladder function and can lead to abnormal urination, urine retention, enuresis, and bladder infections.

Because the Kidneys move fluids in the body, when there's a deficiency, it causes dysfunction of the large intestine, leading to constipation. Deficiency of Kidney yang also causes the Spleen to function poorly, leading to loose stools, undigested food in the stool, anemia, and prolapse. Prolapse is the falling out of place of an organ or body part; the uterus, bladder, and anus are the organs that most commonly prolapse.

WHAT TO AVOID FOR KIDNEY HEALTH

The negative emotions that affect the Kidneys are fear, fright, shock, and anxiety. They make Qi descend, especially in children. In adults, descending Qi can be the root cause of conditions like insomnia and mental restlessness.

When experiencing neck or back pain, and during any other times your Kidneys are out of balance, you'll want to limit the following:

1. SHOCK

Shock means seeing, hearing, or experiencing things that are shocking; for example, receiving a diagnosis of a serious disease like cancer, surviving a car accident, or enduring physical and/or emotional abuse. Those who have experienced war or first-responder situations or anyone who has seen death and destruction firsthand (and who has possibly developed PTSD because of it) is also more likely to suffer from weak Kidneys. Practices like Qigong, journaling, and EFT (Emotional Freedom Technique) are great ways to alleviate shock.

2. OVERWORK

Overwork is the most common cause of depleted Kidney yin. It means mental and physical work for long periods of time, or burning the candle at both ends. One of the ways you may notice your Kidney yin is being depleted is that you will develop what is referred to as "five palm heat." Your hands get red and hot as well as your chest, cheeks, ears, and the tip of your nose.

When I was a butcher and first started building my healing practice, Morning Crane, I averaged four to five hours of sleep several nights a week for four years. I was burning the candle at both ends, and in the late afternoon, my ears and cheeks would turn bright red.

Long work hours, mental overwork, working under harsh conditions, stress, and lack of relaxation all deplete Kidney Qi. Digestion also plays an important role in maintaining healthy Kidney Qi. Improper meals, an irregular eating schedule, eating late at night, discussing business while eating, and not having a balanced exercise routine all contribute to draining this energy as well.

The good news is that yang energy is quickly replenished by post-Heaven Qi, which is why it is so important to eat healthy foods. If you don't, your body starts using up yin essence, which is replenished by sleep. Working too hard and not getting enough sleep also injure the mind, which is another extension of the Kidneys.

3. TOO MUCH SEX

I hate to be the bearer of bad news, but watching too many pornographic movies and having too many orgasms can deplete your Kidney essence. Excessive sexual activity weakens the Kidneys through orgasms because sexual activity is directly related to the Kidney essence. It's not the act of having sex, but the actual release. This includes masturbation. Since the Heart and the Kidneys are closely related, excessive sexual activity can cause heart palpitations and even heart attacks.

An acupuncture teacher once told me a funny and interesting story. She said that the technique called moxibustion was originally developed to preserve the lives of Chinese emperors. Because emperors had many concubines and were having frequent orgasms, they were dying of heart attacks at an early age. They created the moxibustion technique (the burning of mugwort leaves near the skin) for just this scenario, so the emperors could have their fun and still retain some of their Kidney essence!

(An interesting side note—the word *acupuncture* is made up of two Chinese characters, one representing a needle and the other representing moxibustion.)

On the other hand, a Heart deficiency caused by sadness and anxiety weakens the Kidneys and causes impotence or inability to achieve orgasm. The Liver is responsible for the smooth circulation of Qi and blood, particularly in the abdominal region, also referred to as the Lower Burner. Therefore, stagnation of Liver Qi and/or Liver Blood will influence your sexual life and can lead to frigidity, the inability to reach orgasm, or impotence in men. How many orgasms you should have per day or per week depends on your underlying constitution and age. Some clinical textbooks suggest that between the ages of 18 and 25, having seven to eight orgasms per day is okay! As you age, obviously that number goes down.

Don't get me wrong—a healthy sex drive is important for a healthy, balanced life. In fact, if you have a diminished sex drive, it points to a weakness and deficiency inside the body, particularly in the Kidneys. But look at professional boxers, for example. Many fighters will refrain from having an orgasm in the two to four weeks before a fight because they know it weakens their body and can inhibit their energy and performance in the ring. If you want to test out this philosophy, the next time you feel a cold or flu coming on, have multiple orgasms. Chances are, you'll get sicker.

Kidney essence naturally declines with age. In fact, in Chinese medicine, the process of aging is the result of a decrease in Kidney essence. The reason we see a loss of hearing, bone density, sexual function, and memory along with deteriorating teeth and graying hair is because this essence diminishes with age.

The key is to age gracefully. None of us can defy the laws of nature and avoid getting old, but *how* we age depends on how we follow the above guidelines as well as our diet.

BALANCING YOUR WATER ELEMENT

Use these tips to help if your Water element / Kidney system is out of balance:

FENG SHUI BASIC REMEDIES

Place the head of your bed on the north wall of the room. Hang pictures of water in your environment. Adding sounds of water from a fountain or the music of running water will also help. Bowl shapes and hues of blue and black are advantageous. Wearing or painting your room with those colors strengthens the Kidneys. Living near water is also beneficial, as long as it's not too cold and you don't suffer from excessively damp conditions. In feng shui, the ideal place for most people to live, energetically speaking, is halfway up a mountainside with a lake below. The reason is because it creates the proper balance of Fire and Water. The mountain peak represents fire and the lake represents water, which helps us energetically because it's the same way inside the body. The Heart (fire) and Kidneys (water) need to be in proper balance for the body, mind, and spirit to flourish.

GET ENOUGH SLEEP

The primary way the Kidneys rejuvenate is through sleep. Sleep is not just the Kidneys' number one tonic for repair, but our body's as well. Sleep in a cool, dark, quiet room. Try to cut out all light from the window so you'll sleep more soundly. Studies have shown that people tend to sleep better when the room they are in is cooler.

LOWER STRESS

Control your stress levels by getting regular massage and acupuncture. Go for daily walks and get out in nature. Surround yourself with positive and fun people. Avoid environments that cause fear and/or shock. Also, avoid watching things that are violent. Too much of this can rob you of your Kidney Qi.

Three belly laughs per day can also help to lower stress and boost your Kidneys.

RECOMMENDED FOODS

Avoid foods that are salty, greasy, fatty, and fried as well as ice-cold drinks, sugar, and an overconsumption of alcohol. No stimulants—reduce or stop all coffee, chocolate, etc. (a little green tea is okay). All these things weaken the Kidney network and contribute to inflammation.

Eat things that are naturally salty, such as saltwater fish (as long as they aren't too large, like shark), sardines, sea veggies, and seaweed. Eat a pack of seaweed snacks daily.

Eat fruits and vegetables that are blue or black, such as blueberries and blackberries. In winter, make sure you are eating foods that are naturally grown in your area.

Avoid low-fat diets; fats are needed for the production of hormones and for Kidney yin health. Eat fats that are naturally present in nuts and organic animal products. Eat organic butter, ghee, and cheese from grass-fed cows, but in moderation—too much will produce phlegm in the body.

OTHER RECOMMENDATIONS

Avoid wearing wet or cold clothing for too long. The kidneys dislike cold environments, so if you're someone who likes to surf and wear a wetsuit (especially in Northern California where the water is cold), be sure to warm up those kidneys right away by taking off your wet clothing immediately.

- Surround yourself with Water types if you are deficient.

- Practice the Kidney Cleansing Exercise and the healing sound of *fuuu*.

- Develop stronger willpower by practicing positive mantras, prayers, and invocations.

As mentioned earlier, the Kidneys are the root of yin and yang in the body. Therefore, the Kidney diet is broken down into two parts, Kidney yang and Kidney yin deficiency.

HEALING KIDNEY YANG DEFICIENCY

Kidney yang deficiency is characterized by impotence, infertility, coldness, swollen extremities, swollen face, frequent urination, premature ejaculation, diarrhea, low sex drive, low energy, fatigue, pale face and tongue, low back pain, knee pain or weakness, deafness, ringing in the ears, and generally feeling as though the "fire of life" is out.

Foods recommended to help this deficiency include warming foods like chicken, lamb, beef, scallions, sesame seeds, fish, baked tofu, soybeans, walnuts, eggs, lentils, black beans, lotus seeds, a little wine, cinnamon-bark tea, trout, quinoa, anise, fennel, cooked grains, soups, rice, oats, roasted barley, basmati rice, parsnips, sweet potatoes, onions, leeks, pumpkin, squash, carrots, yams, peas, garlic, turnips, stewed fruits, chickpeas, chestnuts, pistachios, liver of lamb/beef/chicken, veal, goat, venison, mackerel, tuna, anchovy, prawns, salmon, mussels, black pepper, fresh or dried ginger, cloves, cinnamon, cardamom, rosemary, turmeric, nutmeg, chives, spring onions, molasses, rice syrup, barley malt, and dates.

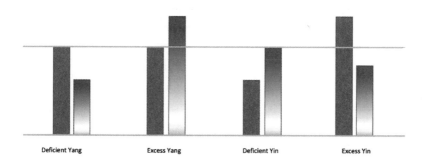

| Deficient Yang | Excess Yang | Deficient Yin | Excess Yin |

HEALING KIDNEY YIN DEFICIENCY

Kidney yin deficiency is characterized by a lack of water to cool the inner fire, manifesting in heat symptoms. These symptoms may include irritability, insomnia, red cheeks, night sweats, low fever in the afternoons, damp palms, damp soles of the feet, dry mouth, low back pain, seminal emission, ringing in the ears, red tongue, and blurry vision. See image above.

Foods recommended to aid this deficiency are energy cooling foods like mulberries, apples, peaches, pears, fresh vegetables, soybeans, tofu, soy sprouts, chrysanthemum flowers, almonds, black beans, mung beans, wheat, oats, rice, millet, barley, almond oil, kelp, spirulina, tofu, tempeh, unsalted pumpkin seeds, unsalted sunflower seeds, adzuki beans, kidney beans, chicken, black-boned chicken, duck, pigeon, eggs, organic bone marrow, Spanish mackerel, sardines, oysters, mussels, clams, cuttlefish, squid, perch, seaweed, eel, bird's nest soup, zucchini, squash, potatoes, sweet potatoes, melons, string beans, beets, button mushrooms, apples, bananas, blueberries, blackberries, mangoes, coconut, olive oil, black sesame seeds, flax seeds, pork, and dairy foods.

Avoid hot foods, spicy foods, smoking, alcohol, stress, and strong emotions (as much as possible).

7

BACK PAIN IN OTHER FIVE ELEMENT TYPES

Although back pain is more common in Wood and Water types, other element types suffer from it as well. If you're an Earth, Metal, or Fire type, this chapter will help you learn the strategies to balance elemental dysfunctions that may be causing your neck and back pain.

THE EARTH ARCHETYPE

If you're an Earth type, you're governed by the Stomach, Spleen, and Pancreas.

When Earth types are in balance, they have strong digestion, a sense of fairness, strong muscles, and a powerful intellect. They are known for being very grounded and centered. When Earth types are out of balance, we see overweight or underweight conditions, weak muscles, digestive problems, excessive phlegm or postnasal drip, overintellectualizing, thinking too much, and anxiety.

The Stomach is responsible for taking the food and fluid we ingest and helping it rot and ripen. It's then sent to the Spleen, where it's further transformed. Finally it's transported up to the chest, where it's used in the production of blood.

Each of the five major organs has certain energies associated with it. I love that the Stomach and Spleen possess the "Designer Qi," called the Gu

Chi (Get it? Gucci?). One of the main functions of the Stomach and Spleen is to take the essence of our food and help turn it into blood.

The energy of all five major organs moves in a certain direction. The energy of the Stomach should descend (not ascend) and the Spleen's energy should ascend to the chest. When this flow is obstructed, disharmony in the Stomach, Spleen, or Liver will affect other related organs as well.

Earth represents stability and harmonizes all other elements. The major physical characteristic of Earth types is plumpness: in the abdominal area, lower cheeks of the face, upper arms, and calves. Earth people tend to be sedentary. They value comfort, consistency, and pleasure. They thoroughly enjoy food and companionship. They are the collectors of the world and love to accumulate possessions and people. Earth people become attached to things and loved ones and have a fondness for sweets and starches. They are often considered warm and affectionate. They feel excessive sympathy for those they care about. As a result, Earth people tend to worry and become overly involved in the lives of others.

When the Earth element is in excess, there is a strong tendency to overeat and gain weight, to the point of obesity. Furthermore, Earth stagnation can affect the circulation of lymphatic fluid. Blood may pool or coagulate, causing such problems as varicose veins, blood clots, and hemorrhoids.

When the Earth element is deficient, you will experience Stomach (digestive) problems. You may struggle to ingest new ideas as well. In addition, you might experience conditions like anorexia, bulimia, diabetes, and flatulence. Earth deficiency is common when you nurture others too much at the expense of yourself. This is thought to be an underlying emotional causal factor in cancer. Earth people move slowly and can get stuck in habits. Movement and change are encouraged for a more balanced Earth element.

The Earth archetype has a pale complexion, strong thighs, and a wide jaw. Earth types should have strong muscles but must take care not to gain weight, because they tend toward large bellies and somewhat heavy bodies. They may not be overly ambitious, but they are calm, generous, and (usually) centered.

Earth types treat people fairly. They can be trusted with carrying out a plan and getting things done. When in balance, Earth people are very centered, but when out of balance, they tend to worry constantly and may be prone to digestive disorders. They also may be susceptible to arthritis if their muscles aren't strong. Earth types make great managers and organizers, although their focus can be weak, making the simultaneous handling of numerous tasks difficult. They respond well to change as long as it is gradual.

The negative emotions that affect the Spleen are pensiveness, worry, and anxiety. The positive virtues are serenity and centeredness. Because of the Spleen's connection to the Earth element, when an Earth type is in balance, positive virtues will be predominant and the presence of negative emotions signals a need to take corrective action. Addressing these early signs of imbalance is key in preventing larger issues down the line. In keeping neck and back pain at bay, it's best to keep a close watch on changes in your emotional well-being.

THE SPLEEN'S FUNCTIONS

Understanding more about the Spleen's functions can help shed light on Earth element imbalances. Because all disease in the body, including pain and inflammation, can be traced back to organ dysfunction, paying particular attention to the role of the Spleen and its presence in the body can allow you to develop a keen awareness of it in your dominant Earth element. This deep understanding and awareness are the foundation for well-being because you will, in turn, develop a greater capacity to respond to your body and its signals.

Chinese medicine's understanding of the Spleen's functions is different from that of Western medicine. Chinese medicine dictates that the Spleen is located in the middle of the body cavity and is the main organ of the digestive system. It is divided into yin (material structure) and yang (the heat necessary to digest food and drink). The Spleen's functions are transporting, distributing, and transforming nutrients; circulating blood within the vessels; and holding the organs in place. It's connected to the muscles, limbs, mouth, and lips. It also controls taste.

The Stomach and Spleen transport, distribute, and transform nutrients. According to Chinese medicine, our food and drink go first to the Stomach, where it and the Spleen digest them. Then the digested matter travels through the pylorus, where it is sent to the small intestine to be transformed into waste. Any food that isn't considered waste is absorbed by the Spleen.

The Spleen is most active between the hours of 9:00 a.m. and 11:00 a.m. and the Stomach is most active between 7:00 a.m. and 9:00 a.m. Therefore, this is the most beneficial time to eat, and breakfast should be the largest meal of the day.

The Spleen produces Qi and blood by using the water and nutrients it absorbs from food and sending them to the Lungs. The Lungs then combine nutrients with the air taken in to help form what is referred to as our "Gathering" Qi. This Qi spreads other Qi and clear fluids to all parts of the body, keeping the *five viscera* (Heart, Lung, Liver, Spleen, and Kidney) nourished.

If the Spleen is not functioning properly, you will notice a lack of appetite, indigestion, fullness and distension in the epigastrium, loose stools, lassitude, weight loss, and other diseases.

The Spleen also absorbs and transports water. If the Spleen cannot absorb water properly and retains it, the result is edema, dampness, phlegm, and diarrhea. The Spleen absorbs food and water at the same time, and both functions are connected, so an abnormal function of one will lead to dysfunction of the other.

HOUSING THE INTELLECT, OR THE YI QI

The Spleen works together with the Stomach and is referred to as our post-Heaven Qi—the energy we create for ourselves by including the right diet, exercise, and spiritual practice in our lives. As stated earlier, each of the five major internal organs of the body is said to house a spiritual component. They are collectively known as the "five souls." The soul of the Spleen houses the intellect or Yi Qi. This soul, or spirit, does not fit the classical definition, but it tells us whether the organ is healthy and in balance or unhealthy and out of balance.

When the Spleen is functioning properly, we're able to reason and understand objectively. The Spleen influences our capacity for thinking, studying, concentrating, focusing, and memorizing. Although other internal organs, like the Heart and Kidneys, also play a role in thinking, it is said that when the Spleen is functioning properly, we are able to concentrate and memorize things more easily. On the other hand, studying or doing mental work that requires concentrating for long periods of time will create a deficiency of the Spleen.

Emotions or tendencies that harm the Spleen and Stomach are worry, anxiety, and overthinking. In addition, you may experience symptoms such as lack of appetite or the inability to digest food properly if the Spleen is not functioning well.

Because of the location of the Spleen, Qi gets knotted when you worry excessively. You may also complain of mid-back pain, as the stagnation of Qi forces pressure onto the ribs.

CONTROLLING BLOOD

The Spleen controls all the blood in the body and keeps it circulating in the vessels. If there is a lack of Qi, blood will not flow normally. When this happens, it can result in blood in the stool, a bloody nose, hemorrhages, bruising easily, or uterine bleeding.

The Spleen plays a crucial role in the development of blood. It extracts the essence from our food and drink and sends it up to the chest, where it forms blood in the Heart in combination with Qi from the Kidneys. Therefore, the Spleen is essential for the formation of Qi and blood. We have a saying that *the blood contains the Qi and Qi moves the blood around the body.* Like yin and yang, one cannot exist without the other.

CONTROLLING THE MOUTH AND LIPS

The mouth is where we take in nourishment. It's also the most sensual part of the face. The size of our mouth shows the size of our appetite. The bigger someone's mouth, the more they want. This relates not only to food but to affection and information as well.

The mouth expresses emotions easily with a smile or a kiss. It is the second-most changeable feature on the face, after the eyes. Most facial expressions require movement of our mouths. The mobility of the muscles around the mouth allows us to change its shape. Unfortunately, most people tend to press their lips together and make them smaller.

The mouth displays a person's generosity and their ability to give. People with a lot of Earth energy have larger mouths. Mouth size is measured in relation to the nose. Create a triangle starting at the center point of the bridge of the nose and follow the sides of the nose in a straight line down to the mouth area. An average mouth is the same length as the base of this imaginary triangle. A mouth that goes beyond this measurement is considered wide. When the corners of the mouth don't reach this distance, the mouth is considered small.

To the ancient Chinese, a large mouth was considered a fortunate feature. Men with large mouths were said to be more capable of attracting a good wife. People with large mouths like to buy many presents for people they love as well as for business associates. They can be known to spontaneously give things even to strangers or new acquaintances. People with average-sized mouths are still generous but are particular about how much they give and to whom. People with small mouths are more conditional about giving and find it difficult to give unless there is a good reason. They give because someone deserves it or because they are expected to give something and do so based on practicality more than emotion.

Lip size is also a factor. Lip fullness is evaluated based on the fleshiness of the rest of the face. Someone whose face is earthier, with plump cheeks and a puffy nose, will have bigger lips. Someone with angular features and taut skin will have thinner lips. Exceptions to this are called "magnified traits." An example of a magnified trait is a large mouth and full lips on a person with a long, thin nose.

In general, fuller lips belong to people who are more emotionally expressive, those who are romantic and sensual. Their lips indicate a desire for pleasure. People with thinner lips are more reserved emotionally, especially if they hold them pressed together.

We can often tell if somebody overly nurtures other people and doesn't get enough back for themselves by what are referred to as "smoker's lines" (vertical lines above the upper lip). People who smoke develop these lines from continually pursing their lips. They are, in essence, trying to nurture themselves (even though smoking is not a healthy way to do that). But smoker lines are also seen in nonsmokers who give most of their Earth energy to others and don't get enough back in return.

You can tell the Spleen is deficient as well if they complain of having a sweet taste in their mouth or if they have pale lips and facial tone. If there's too much heat in the Stomach and Spleen, the lips will tend to be dried and cracked.

CONTROLLING THE RISE OF QI

Regarding the internal organs, most people would agree that they sit where they sit because God placed them there! They're not wrong. There is something much greater than all of us that created the human body and all living organisms.

The Spleen is the main organ responsible for helping raise Qi and holding our internal organs in place. Anatomically, abdominal muscles and tissues, such as the mesentery, are responsible for this function. Since the Spleen controls these tissues, if it is weak, they will be unable to do their job and organs will fall out of place. When this happens, it's called a prolapse. The most common prolapses are of the anus, uterus, and bladder. We can fix these conditions pretty easily with application of various Qigong practices that strengthen the Stomach and Spleen while reducing worry and anxiety and by changing the diet to specifically strengthen Spleen and Stomach functions.

Another example of Qi rising is the ability to hold blood within its vessels. For example, we can tell that the Spleen is weak in a young child who suddenly develops chronic nosebleeds. If asked, he or she might state that they're worried about starting at a new school or moving to a new town. This excess of worry and anxiety causes blood to fall out of the blood vessels, leading to nosebleeds. The Spleen also raises Qi when it separates the pure essence from food and drink and sends it up to the chest, not only to be made into blood but also to nourish the space between the skin and muscles.

CONTROLLING THE MUSCLES AND LIMBS

In my clinical practice, Spleen dysfunctions are some of the most common conditions we see. Problems are caused by overtaxing the mind with excessive mental work or worries, eating things that harm the Stomach and Spleen, and doing unrelated activities while eating.

The nourishing essence produced by Spleen Qi is distributed to the forelimbs as well as the muscles and tissues. In fact, if you are an Earth type, you should have strong muscles or the ability to gain muscle mass quicker than other element typologies. If your Spleen is weak, you may tend to have flabby muscles; this is evidenced by dangling triceps, for example. You may suffer from overweight or underweight conditions. Your abdomen will be loose and you may have weak muscles or feel tired. In severe cases, you could suffer from atrophy.

Another way to tell that the Spleen is weak is if a person drags their feet when they walk. This occurs because the muscles of the legs are too weak to properly lift the feet off the ground.

BALANCING DEFICIENCIES IN YOUR EARTH ELEMENT

FENG SHUI BASIC REMEDIES

Yellow, orange, and earth tones support the Earth element. To benefit this element, hang pictures of flatlands or plains in your home and office. The Earth element is represented by architecture that is flat and square. Having your surroundings made of "earth," which includes brick or even concrete, is positive for supporting Earth, as is including square-shaped sculptures in your environment.

If you are deficient in the Earth element and especially if you have dampness, the ideal place to live would be in the Southwest. Arizona, Southern California, and New Mexico are optimal locations, as is having a house made of brick with a flat roof.

DIET AND LIFESTYLE RECOMMENDATIONS

Avoid foods with excessive amounts of sugar. Foods that can help relieve fatigue due to weakness are yams, corn, and certain types of rice. In addition, people who need to balance out their Earth element will greatly benefit from Qigong practices that help root Qi as well as those that harmonize the Stomach and Spleen.

THE METAL ARCHETYPE

If you took the Five Element Questionnaire and discovered you are a Metal type, you are governed by the Lungs. Chances are you have a long, thin nose and a triangular face and you like the finer things in life. You may prefer the color white or gray tones. Because having Metal as your dominant element will impact the way imbalances show up and how you can address them, it is important to have a deep understanding of what makes a Metal-dominant person unique and how a Metal nature will show up in the body. As with the other elements, the entire system benefits when it's kept in balance and addressing the root causes of imbalance is the first step in healing your neck and back pain.

As a Metal type, you may hide your sadness because it's not the face you want to show to the world. When you're out of balance, you may catch colds more easily, find that your voice is softer than usual, or feel weaker than normal. You may also become more prone to conditions like eczema and asthma.

The main features of Metal archetypes are small bones, fair skin, angular features, and broad shoulders. Metal is an element of duality, or opposites: Metal people are visionaries and idealists, yet they are practical. They love both luxury and simplicity. They are very sensitive. They are often seen as aloof and distant, but that's because they need to maintain boundaries or they will get easily overwhelmed. Metal types are particular and perfectionistic. They are especially prone to health problems involving boundary violations.

Metal types have strong immune systems. They can get sick frequently but recover quickly. They often develop skin and respiratory system allergies early in life, including hives, eczema, and asthma. Metal types also get sunburned easily and prefer staying indoors. They are more readily bitten by mosquitoes because of their ability to release a large quantity of carbon dioxide through the breath as they detoxify their Lungs. Metal people prefer to cocoon in what they consider safe environments, with a minimum of dust or clutter and a maximum of beauty and stylish design.

When people develop certain types of allergies later in life, they have become Metal deficient. This also applies to those who never had respiratory ailments as children but suffer from them frequently as adults. Other signs of Metal deficiency are slow-healing skin, a weakened immune system, and chronic respiratory or skin conditions such as recurring bronchitis, emphysema, and psoriasis.

Excessive accumulations of phlegm that cause chronic coughing and shortness of breath are associated with Metal stagnation. Tuberculosis and leprosy, which are conditions of stagnation, occur because of unclean, overcrowded environments. The Metal element type is more mental than physical and requires refinement, cleanliness, tranquility, and space to thrive.

Metal types are rational, independent, and strong-willed. They normally have a strong, loud voice because their Lungs are their most powerful attribute.

Metal types can be either positive or destructive, depending on their intent. They have the ability to gather others for a positive cause or a negative outcome. They are aggressive in pursuing goals. They are emotional, confident, and intuitive, but at the same time are often unwilling to express their true inner feelings.

A negative aspect of Metal types is that they may isolate themselves, withdrawing from activities and society in general. Metal's negative attributes are grief, sorrow, and sadness.

The Metal type has a strongly built body, with broad and square shoulders. They tend to walk slowly, pushing their chest out with their shoulders back. Metal represents courage, righteousness, justice, and truth.

THE LUNGS' FUNCTIONS

The Metal element relates to the Lungs and large intestine, thus controlling the immune system. The related tissues are hair, skin, and the nose, which controls the sense of smell. Addressing symptoms of imbalance in these areas of the body will assist in reestablishing balance in the Metal element. The Lungs are most active between 3:00 a.m. and 5:00 a.m., and the Large Intestine is most active between 5:00 a.m. and 7:00 a.m. The Lungs are most prone to disease during autumn months and they decline in the climatic condition of dryness. If they stay in harmony, Metal-dominant individuals maintain greater health, avoiding larger issues like disease, pain, and inflammation. If you are a Metal type and are experiencing neck and back pain, take a look at the element's qualities and what you can do to bring yourself back into flow.

The Lungs are made up of two lobes and connect to the larynx, bronchi, and trachea, ultimately opening into the nose. They are divided into the yin of the Lung (material structure) and the Qi of the Lung (functions); the term "yang of the Lung" is rarely used. The Lungs are considered the most superficial organ of the body because of their relationship to the nose and their responsibility for regulating the opening and closing of pores in the skin (which makes them the body's most external organ).

Lungs have to work directly with the Kidneys and the Spleen (see image below). For us to inhale, the Kidneys need to be able to grasp air from the Lungs and pull it down. When we exhale, the Lungs grasp the moisture from the Kidneys, not only to moisten the Lungs but to aid in the dispersing function.

Origin, Transformation and Excretion of Blood and Fluids

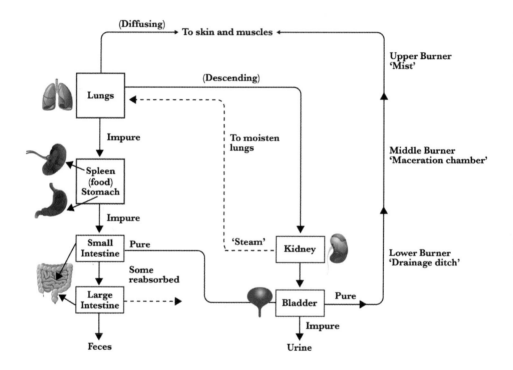

TAKING CHARGE OF QI

The Lungs exchange air between the interior and the exterior of the body. The exchanging of carbon dioxide for oxygen enables our cellular metabolism to function smoothly. If the Lungs are harmed by external pathogenic factors, this gas exchange becomes difficult.

CONTROLLING THE DEFENSIVE QI

Aside from the Lungs, the Spleen, Kidneys, lymphatic system, and Liver all play a crucial role in our immune function. The Lungs house our Defensive Qi, also referred to as the Wei Qi, which protects us from the intrusion of pathogens. This Defensive Qi is like an energetic bubble that surrounds all of us.

It is said that there are three levels of Wei Qi. The first level resides two to three inches above the surface of the body and relates to our physical selves. The second resides two to three feet around the body and relates to the mental/emotional aspects of our being. The third level resides several feet around the body and connects to our spiritual aspects.

When people say, "Chris, I don't have an energetic bubble around me!" I assure them that they've experienced this Wei Qi at some point in their lives. Say somebody walks up behind you and you don't see them or hear them but you "feel" them. That person has walked into your Wei Qi. If you sense someone staring at you or see that somebody is watching you from four car lanes over, that's because they are tapping into your Wei Qi.

Generally speaking, when our immune systems are healthy and vibrant, our energetic bubbles can extend farther. What tends to happen when our immunity is deficient, especially during autumn when the Lungs are at their weakest, is that this bubble moves closer to the skin. This sets us up for the possibility of catching viruses during the cold and flu season.

It is said that our Defensive Qi flows underneath the skin as well. When it's healthy, a person's immune system will be strong. However, if the Lungs are weak due to excessive work, poor diet, extreme grief and sadness, or being stooped over a desk, it can mean we are more susceptible to illness.

OPERATING THE QI OF THE WHOLE BODY

The Lungs spread Qi, nutrients from food, and fluid to nourish the body, skin, and hair; warm the muscles; and help maintain normal water metabolism. The Lungs are also responsible for forming the Zong Qi, or Gathering Qi, of the chest. Inhaled air and the essence of foods we eat mix and accumulate in the chest to form Zong Qi. This Qi leaves from the larynx and promotes the Lungs' respiratory activities. It spreads through the body through Heart channels and warms the viscera, bowels, and tissues.

The Lungs control both the ascending and the descending Qi of the body. If they are not functioning properly, the ascending and descending of Qi is adversely affected and shows up as shortness of breath, tiredness, a quiet voice, and drowsiness.

When the Lungs are not in proper alignment and are therefore not cleaning the air they take in, Qi cannot spread from the Lungs throughout the body. This shows up as coughing, asthma, and a stuffy sensation in the chest. If the Lungs are functioning properly, they are able to spread water to the Kidneys and urinary bladder, thus smoothing the metabolism of water. If water does not flow smoothly to the Kidneys and urinary bladder, it results in dysuria (difficult or painful urination), edema, and phlegm-retention diseases.

The Lungs have two functions, dispersing Qi and causing Qi to descend. The dispersing of Qi and descending of Qi both oppose and support each other. If the Lungs cannot disperse Qi, it cannot descend and vice versa. This relationship maintains normal airflow and Qi.

BEING ASSOCIATED WITH THE SKIN AND HAIR

The Lungs supply the skin and hair with the fluids they need to stay moist and bright. When the skin is healthy, it can defend the body from outside pathogens. If the Lungs are not dispersing fluids properly, the result is profuse sweating, vulnerability to the common cold, dry skin, and withered or dry hair.

CONNECTING TO THE NOSE

We can tell how good someone's stamina is by looking at the sides of their nose. If Lung Qi is strong, the nose will be open. Respiration will be easy, and the sense of smell will be strong. We can tell a person has too much heat in their Lungs if their nostrils are flared and red. Because the nose relates to the Lungs and the Metal element, this area tells us a lot about how well someone spends or invests their money. You can tell by the size of the nostrils how giving or stingy a person is with their money and their energy. The nose will tell us if they are shrewd, power hungry, or resistant to authority or have the potential for high or low blood sugar. If someone complains of a metallic taste in their mouth, it could be a sign that their Lung Qi is deficient. If they experience a rank smell in their breath, it usually means they are suffering from a chronic retention of phlegm.

HOUSING THE CORPOREAL SOUL

Recall that according to Chinese medicine, each of the five major organs is governed by a different soul.

The Lungs are governed by the Corporeal Soul, which is the most physical and material part of a human's soul. When it's healthy, it helps our physical being. This is the part of the soul that returns to Earth at the time of death. You could say that it's the somatic, or bodily, manifestation of the soul.

This is where our attachments to people or worldly possessions come in. It is said that ghosts are created when a person's energy is too heavy and unable to ascend to Heaven because of a strong connection to a person or possession in this physical world.

The Corporeal Soul is affected by all emotions but especially by disappointment, grief, shame, guilt, and sadness. These emotions are associated with and stem from the inability to deal with loss, manifesting as repressed grief and sorrow.

This part of the soul is also known as the animal soul. It controls our primal instincts and can be seen in the body's basic physiological functioning. However, it can also be looked at in relation to our physical and material needs, as in collecting and holding on to what is needed to survive. This is discernment, where instinct and judgment occur within and in relation to the surrounding world. Another trait of the animal soul is the ability to feel emotion and pain without dwelling on experiences.

When the Corporeal Soul is out of balance, we see conditions like asthma. Holding on to the belongings of deceased family or friends can keep grief alive and weaken the Lungs. Keeping the urn of ashes of a deceased loved one in your bedroom can disrupt not only your sleep but your spirit. If you're not getting enough sleep, the Kidneys will be weakened, which will in turn weaken the Lungs. Going to too many open-casket funerals or holding on to gifts and pictures from a past breakup can also disrupt the Corporeal Soul. Having these kinds of attachments is a sign that your Corporeal Soul is out of balance.

BALANCING METAL DEFICIENCIES

FENG SHUI BASIC REMEDIES

If your dominant element is Metal, keeping it in balance is key to maintaining physical health. To support the Metal element, include metal items and furnishings in your life and house. Use a lot of white or silver. Decorate your house with arched, curved, or semicircular furnishings to gather more Metal energy. In architecture, domed metal roofs and structures made primarily of metal attract Metal energy.

From a feng shui standpoint, place the head of your bed facing west and use white, silver, and/or gray tones in your bedroom. Put a metal wind chime outside your window and hang pictures or sculptures of dome-shaped objects.

If you tend to catch colds or flu easily, it could be a sign of a weak Metal element. See the next couple of sections for additional tips that will help restore balance.

WHAT TO AVOID

If your Metal element is out of balance, avoid foods that are greasy, fatty, or fried. Sugar, ice-cold drinks, and all processed foods should be eliminated. If you crave those foods, it's a sign that organs other than the Lungs are out of balance and are contributing to the situation. The craving of pungent foods, like garlic or onions, is a signal from the body that the Lungs are out of balance and need help.

If you crave salt, that's your Kidneys talking to you, letting you know that they're part of the root cause of the imbalance. Try to avoid dry environments, especially ones with a draft.

Suppressing feelings of loss or grief is bad for Lung health. If you are a Metal type, you desire to express yourself and be heard.

Avoid contaminated environments where the air isn't clean. Avoid smoking or being in smoky environments. Also, if you are around people who are in a continual state of sadness, you can pick up on that energy and it will affect your Lung Qi.

DIET AND LIFESTYLE RECOMMENDATIONS

Eat foods that are white and/or pungent, such as onions, fennel, leeks, cinnamon, garlic, and ginger. Cordyceps, reishi, and shiitake mushrooms are great for building Lung Qi. Another perk of these common foods is that you can buy them in extract or pill form (but eating them in food form is preferred).

Astragalus root is also helpful for Lung Qi, as is another traditional herbal formula that you can buy online called Jade Windscreen. Both astragalus root and Jade Windscreen help build Lung strength, which is especially important going into the cold and flu season.

Allow yourself to be heard, open yourself up to being vulnerable, and show your tears when you're sad. Let go of worldly attachments and anything that holds you back from being as free as the wind.

THE FIRE ARCHETYPE

If your Five Element Questionnaire score shows that you are primarily a Fire type, your strength lies in the blood and blood vessels. In nature, Fire is responsible for warming and achieving clarity. A Fire type can illuminate and provide comfort in any situation. They are leaders who are highly charismatic and self-driven. They are deeply passionate motivators. The Fire type enjoys being in the limelight. They are adventurous and excited by change. This can bring about great success—or failure if they're not careful.

This archetype tends to walk fast unless the Spleen is out of balance. Fire people are creative and take on many challenges, which makes them ideal warriors. The Fire type is normally unconcerned with wealth but is fond of beauty. They may have a reddish face with a large nose and curly hair—or lack thereof! They are energetic, active, and like to open themselves to love, which also opens them up to being hurt because they tend to have poor boundaries.

The Fire element relates to the Heart and Small Intestine. The Heart is most active between the hours of 11:00 a.m. and 1:00 p.m., and the Small Intestine is most active between 1:00 and 3:00 p.m. The Pericardium and the Triple Burner belong in the Fire element category as well. The Pericardium is most active between 7:00 and 9:00 p.m. and the Triple Burner from 9:00 to 11:00 p.m.

The Triple Burner is not an actual physiological organ. Think of it as the network that enables all the organs to communicate and function properly (our internal organs are interdependent, not independent).

The Upper Burner can be compared to the "mist." This is where the blood and Qi of the body are produced. The Middle Burner is considered the "maceration chamber" where our food and drink enters the stomach and digestion occurs. The Lower Burner is like a drainage ditch where waste from our food and drink enters the intestines and bladder.

The pericardium is the protective tissue of the Heart. Generally, external pathogenic factors such as high fever, coma, and certain viruses affect the pericardium before they affect the Heart. Although the Heart tends to absorb the brunt of all other negative emotions, those feelings pass through the pericardium first. The Heart houses the primary negative emotions of abandonment, loneliness, and overexcitation (or excess joy) in addition to the positive virtue of love.

FIRE ELEMENT TRAITS

Like the preceding elements, the Fire element has a unique impact on the body and the self. Developing greater awareness of these traits and characteristics expands not only self-knowledge but also an understanding of how the element shows up in the body, giving us the insight and tools we need to return to harmony when the Fire element is thrown off balance. For Fire types, establishing equilibrium of the element is key to eliminating disease, pain, and inflammation in the body.

The major physical signs of Fire are slim hips and shoulders, although some have an hourglass or pear-shaped body. Fire types tend to talk with their hands and have sparkling eyes. They may have redness in the throat or neck areas and have very lively personalities. Their main goal in life is to play. Fire types love new experiences and communicating, whether verbally, with body language, or through their eyes. They are changeable and scattered, charismatic and charming. They tend to flourish in warmer climates and may be drawn to wearing clothes that are pink or red. Fire people are full of ideas and prefer starting over finishing. They enjoy excitement and can become thrill seekers. Fire types are naturally attuned to rhythm and love to dance to a strong beat. They are fun, lively, charming, cute, and playful and are often the life of the party.

Their biggest health problems come from inflammation (such as in lupus, rheumatoid arthritis, and heart disease), which is caused by unrestrained Fire and an overactive nervous system. Fire people are prone to disturbances in speaking and thinking, especially when under pressure. This can be caused by the misfiring of the brain and an overactive imagination. Because the Heart is said to house the mind, if there is a disturbance, you often see conditions such as stuttering, phobias, and mental illness.

The Fire element's primary organ is the Heart, which controls and regulates the expression or suppression of all emotions. Suppression of emotions can therefore cause problems with the Heart, including arrhythmia, atrial fibrillation, tachycardia, depression, and heart disease.

Fire people maintain a youthful persona and try to continue living an erratic life that causes burnout and ultimately sadness. And just like a wildfire, Fire people tend to burn bright and burn out quickly. If you're with a Fire type, it's recommended that you give them time and space to rekindle their spark.

The strength of Fire is reflected in the eyes as well as the tips and corners of all the features and in every marking on the face. Because the Heart is considered emperor, it rules the expression of all emotions. Every organ has its own emotions, but the Heart decides whether the emotion is expressed and how much. The Fire element governs communication of all kinds, especially the use of words spoken verbally or in sign language. Because Fire features show up in the eyes' luster and brightness, you can say that someone who communicates expressively with their eyes is tapping into their Fire element. Also, because the Heart controls expression, facial wrinkles can demonstrate how much expression or repression has been engaged in over time.

Fire can be a dangerous element when overused. It dries up our essence, also referred to as *Jing*, and wears out the body. It's in our nature to play; we need to enjoy life. But if someone habitually plays too much it can become harmful, creating physical and emotional problems.

The negative emotions particularly associated with the Heart are overexcitation, mania, feelings of abandonment, loneliness, sadness, and excessive joy. People often ask me how excessive joy can be dangerous. The reality is that anything that is excessive shows up as disease. Believe it or not, you can actually die of a heart attack from laughing too hard! Think about it. After a laughing attack, the first thing everybody does is sigh or try to catch their breath. That's your Heart's way of trying to regain balance. Also, sadness is often classified as a Heart emotion. Because the Heart and Lungs are so connected, sadness can turn into sorrow, which is a Lung emotion. That then turns to grief, another Lung emotion. And because of this close interconnectedness, these emotions will, in turn, affect the Heart directly.

Chinese face reading says that the two most changeable features on the face are the lips and the eyes. The lips relate to the Earth element and the eyes to the Fire element. The eyes are best at showing emotion. Since there is a complex network of muscles surrounding them, they are the most expressive feature on the face and the most easily marked. This is why as we age, we see lines around the eyes.

We learn early in life how to communicate with our eyes. They speak a silent kind of language. That's why the eyes are so fascinating. The size of our eyes represents the openness of our Heart. They are measured in terms of vertical height and should be viewed in proportion to the rest of the face. For example, someone with large eyes will tend to be more emotional, spontaneous, and dramatic. They may even blurt out things at inappropriate times in public. People with small, squinty eyes tend to be more reserved with their Heart emotions and may be self-critical or critical of others. Many times they are distrustful and become stuck in their heads.

The Fire element rules the firing of the brain's neurons, synapses, and receptor sites. One of the most important aspects of the Fire element is the light of the eyes, called the Shen, or the spirit. You can determine how quick someone's mind is by watching the alertness in their eyes. Babies with bright eyes are recognized as being highly intelligent. The spirit in their eyes shows changes in emotion from moment to moment, and this light also demonstrates how well their nervous system is functioning.

THE HEART'S FUNCTIONS

The Heart is located in the chest slightly to the left. In Chinese medicine, it is believed that the Heart is the most important organ, as it controls the other internal organs and the bowels. The Heart is divided into yin and yang. The yin refers to blood controlled by the Heart and the yang to its actual function as well as the heat and Qi of the Heart. Its main functions are controlling blood circulation, taking charge of mental activities, producing sweat as the fluid of the Heart, housing our consciousness and spirit, and being connected with the tongue and the complexion of the face.

HOUSING THE MIND (SPIRIT—SHEN)

We have a saying that "the Heart houses the mind, which in turn houses Shen, our spirit." According to Chinese medicine, Shen is composed of the complex mental faculties as well as the spiritual aspects of the whole human being. This includes the spiritual components of all the other internal organs: the Corporeal Soul of the Lungs, the Ethereal Soul of the Liver, the intellect of the Spleen, and the willpower of the Kidneys.

For many years, scientists have tried to locate the mind. It's been virtually impossible because the mind itself is a form of Qi and does not reside in the brain. Now there is a group of scientists in California that has developed a system called HeartMath that is proving that our true consciousness resides in the Heart. What does this mean? It means that our Hearts are the center of our awareness and our brain reflects our reality.

In fact, because Fire touches certain features on the face (described below), you can tell the strength of a person's spirit by looking at their eyes. The more intact their spirit, the brighter and more glistening the eyes will be. Those suffering from mental illness tend to have dull, lackluster eyes, and the more dull or lackluster the eyes, the more serious the mental condition.

The Heart controls our mental activities and is responsible for insight and cognition. That's why it is considered the emperor or empress of the body. When Heart functions are normal, a person will have healthy consciousness and mental activities. Abnormalities like insanity, mania, forgetfulness, and bipolar conditions may be brought on by insufficiency of blood, an obstruction of the Heart caused by phlegm and deficiency of Heart Fire.

GOVERNING BLOOD

Blood is formed through three essential organs: the essence from the Kidneys combined with the air we breathe through our Lungs and the food essence derived from the Spleen—all of which are sent up to the chest. The Heart governs blood by transforming our food essence and is one of the organs responsible for circulation. The connection between the Heart and blood is important because it shows the strength of one's overall constitution. Although the underlying constitution is said to be housed in the Kidneys, if Heart blood is deficient, a person will have a weak constitution and will lack strength. On the other hand, if the Heart blood is strong and circulation is good, a person will be full of vigor.

CONTROLLING BLOOD CIRCULATION

Since the Heart governs blood, it naturally controls the vessels through which blood flows. These blood vessels are linked to the Heart, creating a closed system. The Heart's Qi keeps it beating and sends blood through the vessels. When Qi is plentiful, the Heart can maintain a normal rate and strength. The pulse can tell you if Qi is sufficient and whether the blood of the Heart is sufficient. If Heart blood is stagnant, blood vessels will feel hard, and this may lead to issues like coronary artery disease.

CONTROLLING SWEAT, THE FLUID OF THE HEART

Bodily fluid is the most important component of the blood, and sweat comes from this fluid. Sweat is an extension of blood, so profuse sweating means the Heart is using a lot of blood and Qi, which may result in palpitations and a sensation of violent beating in the chest. In addition, too much sweating—from excessive exercise or from cutting weight like we see in wrestling, martial arts, and boxing—hurts the yang of the Heart because so much bodily fluid is lost. This can cause a deficiency of blood, which can lead to anemia. Those who have a yin deficiency in the Heart (yin being the cooling aspect of the body) are likely to sweat at night.

CONNECTING TO THE TONGUE AND FACE

We can see the Heart's condition on the tongue and face because of the large number of blood vessels in each. A bright red face and tongue show that the Heart is functioning well. If the face and tongue are pale and white, the Heart is not functioning optimally, and this may indicate a deficiency of blood. Heart stagnation can be seen in a blue face and a dark purple tongue.

Although the hair on the head is an extension of the Kidneys, it needs the blood's nourishment. Thus, the hair on your head can be a window into the Heart's health. Healthy hair means a healthy Heart.

If the Heart and blood are strong, a person will speak with clearly articulated words and sentences. If there is a blockage or deficiency in the Heart and/or blood, we may see conditions like stuttering, slurred speech, and a sudden inability to talk. In fact, one form of diagnosis in Chinese medicine is looking at the tongue to discern the state of the internal organs as well as present conditions or pathogens. The tip of the tongue connects to the Heart, and by looking at it we can tell if someone is going through emotional distress. For example, if you developed a cold sore on the tip of your tongue, it would indicate an accumulation of heat in the Heart, and therefore it would be a good idea to take inventory of what had recently affected you emotionally.

POINTED TIPS ON THE FACE

Besides the lines of your face, the Fire element shows up in the tips and corners of other features on the face. For example, if someone has very pointed ears, it can indicate extreme ups and downs in their emotional state. If you see a line bisecting the earlobe, it can mean that the person has burned the candle at both ends for too long. This can be a sign of Heart or Kidney disease.

Earlier in this section, we talked about how the Heart connects to the tongue and influences speech. If a person has a very pointed inner canthus of the eye, they likely have a sharp tongue. So if you know someone with a pointed inner canthus, this can be a warning that the closer that person gets to you and the more they know about you, the more likely they are to use what they know to hurt you. The sharper the canthus, the sharper the tongue!

Even though the nose connects to the Metal element and the Lungs, the tip of the nose correlates to the Heart. For example, if you have a line that bisects both nostrils, this shows either the potential for mitral valve prolapse or the possibility of high or low blood pressure. I've found throughout my years of clinical practice that this line is normally present in people with the potential for low blood pressure. If you see a line that cuts horizontally above the tip of the nose, it indicates someone who has suffered a broken Heart that has not been fully dealt with.

BALANCING DEFICIENT FIRE

People who are deficient in the Fire element may be prone to heart-related problems and/or problems with their veins, arteries, and blood. Because the circulatory system impacts all other organs, reestablishing balance in the Fire element is of utmost importance for maintaining physical health. If not addressed and corrected, these issues will create further imbalance in related systems of the body, leading to disease, chronic pain, and inflammation.

If you are deficient in the Fire element or if you're a Fire type who has deviated from your typology, the following are some simple remedies that will help you increase the Fire in your life.

FENG SHUI BASIC REMEDIES

Those who have Fire deficiencies may want to add things into their environment such as candles, things colored red or pink, and pictures depicting fire. Buildings with steep roofs, like church steeples, also help build the element. It is beneficial to add triangular or pyramid shapes to your environment as well. If you are completely deficient in Fire, living on a mountain range with steep peaks or being in a warmer climate will support more of the element's aspects.

WHAT TO AVOID

As a Fire type, it should be your normal tendency to lead with your Heart; therefore, you should strive to express your emotions and not hold them in. Try not to isolate yourself, but give yourself time to recharge. Don't put yourself in a position where your Fire energy is being suppressed, whether in a work environment or in a relationship.

Avoid greasy, fatty, fried foods, smoking, excessive alcohol, too many spicy foods, sugar, and drugs.

DIET AND LIFESTYLE RECOMMENDATIONS

The Heart likes foods that are bitter; for example, kale, apricot kernels, dandelion root and greens, salad greens, endive, burdock root, borage, honeysuckle, forsythia, gardenia, gentian, goldenseal, plantain, echinacea, rhubarb root, and taro root. Though not necessarily bitter, foods that are red can nourish the Heart, especially when there is a yang deficiency or loss of Fire/

heat in the body. Some beneficial red foods are beets, tomatoes, cherries, red beans, watermelon, apples, strawberries, and beef.

You can also add small amounts of bitter herbs like dong quai, chamomile, and milk thistle to your daily diet.

Journal daily and write about how you feel. Develop your voice, and don't allow people to suppress you. Establish strong boundaries with others because they may want to sneak in using methods that tap into or manipulate your Heart chakra, or middle Tan Tien. Laugh often and surround yourself with people who are lighthearted yet loving and caring.

PART TWO

YOUR EASY GUIDE

TO ENDING

BACK PAIN

8

LOW BACK PAIN
AND RELATED CONDITIONS

If you picked up this book because you're experiencing lower back pain and are looking for immediate relief, take heart. This chapter will give you exactly what you're looking for.

If you already have a diagnosis, here's what to do:

- Start with the standard ice/heat protocol (check out the section starting on page 130 titled "The Top Three Remedies to Start Immediately").

- Read the description of your condition in the "Remedies for Common Low-Back Conditions" section and check for specific do-it-yourself (DIY) recommendations. Add those to your daily routine.

- Finally, move on to the longer-term lifestyle recommendations in the "Low Back Pain Maintenance and Prevention" section.

If you're not sure exactly what condition(s) you have, or if you'd like more information about any of them:

- Start with the standard ice/heat protocol.

- Read the description of each condition in the "Remedies for Common Low-Back Conditions" section. Make note of any specific techniques recommended for your symptoms.

- Do the "Top Three Remedies to Start Immediately."

- Incorporate the specific techniques recommended for your condition, if applicable.

- Finally, add to your regimen the recommended longer-term lifestyle recommendations in the "Low Back Pain Maintenance and Prevention" section.

As soon as you can, but definitely once you've started to see some improvement, begin implementing the recommendations in the maintenance and prevention section. This section will give you the tools you need to get stronger and healthier in general, heal your back pain specifically, and, most important, prevent it from recurring in the future.

Ready to dive in? Let's start with the three most important actions you can take right now.

THE TOP THREE REMEDIES TO START IMMEDIATELY

All low back issues have the same root cause and basic care protocol. Any variations to these remedy strategies will be based on your symptoms. You can find these variations listed beneath each condition in the "Remedies for Common Low Back Conditions" section. For details on each remedy, see the following remedies section.

But no matter what your low back challenge is, start with these top three techniques. Do them not just for immediate relief but as fundamental daily practices for ongoing maintenance. The first remedy that many health professionals recommend is ice, but I recommend alternating ice and heat.

1.   STANDARD ICE/HEAT PROTOCOL

If you have low back pain, your practitioner may tell you to ice your lower back. My own past severe back problems started me on my journey with Chinese medicine over 30 years ago. In my experience, lower back pain was exacerbated when I applied ice to it. So I recommend alternating between ice and heat to see which one feels best to you.

If it's a recent injury, then yes, go ahead and ice it. But if it's an older injury or back problem, alternate between ice and heat to see which one feels better. Listen to your body. If you notice that applying heat to the lower back is creating more pain, then stop. If you notice that ice is creating more pain, stop.

Another remedy you may want to try is putting ice on the lower lumbar and heat on the upper back at the same time. With the ice on your lower back, place a heating pad on your thoracic spine between the shoulder blades and opposite the heart. Then alternate the heat and ice every 15 minutes or so. For example, you'd do 15 minutes of ice on the lower lumbar and heat on the upper back, then switch to 15 minutes of ice on the upper back and heat on the lower lumbar. Do this technique at least two to three times per day. Then walk for about five minutes afterward.

The most important thing is to listen to your body and stop any technique that makes you more uncomfortable.

No injury, or still feeling the effects of an old injury? Then move on to these tried-and-true DIY methods and start feeling relief today.

2.   PSOAS STRETCH

There are some yoga and Pilates poses that can help you stretch your psoas, but in my experience, nothing works as well as this exercise. It is best done daily. See image below.

- Lie on a massage table, coffee table, workout bench or other type of bench, or two hard chairs with no arms set side by side.

- Bring your buttocks to the edge of the table, bench, or chairs.

- Dangle your left leg off the edge, then bring your right knee to your chest.

- Rotate the right knee across your body, internally rotating the femur bone and drawing the knee toward the left shoulder.

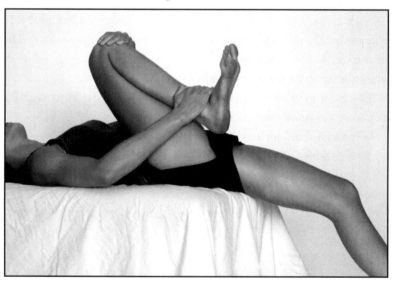

When this stretch is done correctly, you'll feel a pinching or burning sensation on the right hip crease and on the top of the right thigh, which indicates that the psoas is engaged. You may or may not feel a slight pulling or stretch on the left thigh. Take some deep breaths and hold the position for 30 to 60 seconds.

Then switch and do the same thing on the other side. Finally, get up and walk back and forth for one or two minutes.

Key Points

Don't be alarmed if you notice some pinching or burning sensations in your back. This is normal because the psoas is at the root of back issues and connects to the spine. As you open up and stretch this muscle, the pain will dissipate. See images below

Don't use your bed or the floor. A bed is too soft and the floor does not give you the correct angle for the dangling leg. You need gravity to help with hip extension.

Movement is the key to prevention of disease. Therefore, the more you walk after doing this stretch, the better and faster it will heal.

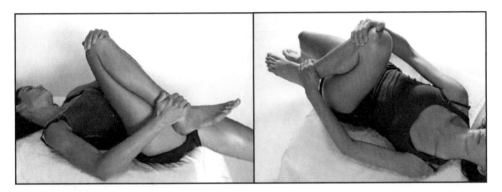

For a demonstration of the psoas stretch, scan the below QR code.

3.   GALLBLADDER PRESS

This technique is best administered by someone else because they will have better leverage, but you can still do it yourself and get some benefit. See image below.

Lie face up on a hard surface with your right knee bent, right foot flat on the floor, and left leg extended straight out.

With your right hand, find the top of the right hip bone (GB 27 and GB 28 acupoints). Press on the inside of your hip bone toward the groin and thigh crease (inguinal groove) with your second, third, and fourth fingers.

Once you're pressing on the top of the right hip bone, begin to curl the fingers laterally toward the inner hip and outer thigh.

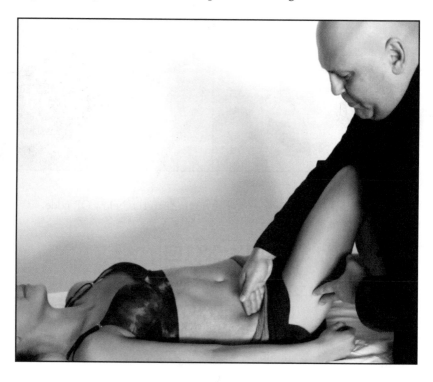

Press and hold for 30 to 45 seconds. Apply as much pressure as possible. It will be uncomfortable. See images on the next page.

Then, maintaining the same amount of pressure, extend the right leg until it's flat on the floor. Meanwhile, the left leg stays flat the whole time.

Switch and do the same thing on the left side. Then walk for one or two minutes, just like you did after the psoas stretch.

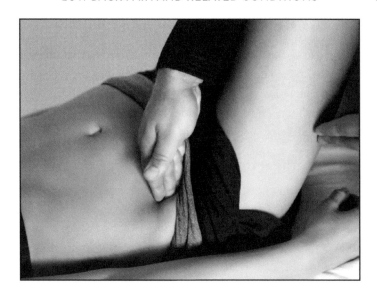

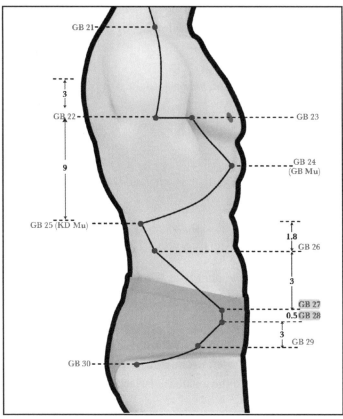

DIY REMEDIES: YOUR EASY GUIDE

After you've read the descriptions above, follow these instructions to relieve your pain ASAP. Then continue to apply the remedies for your condition as ongoing maintenance.

Below are additional recommendations for general low back pain followed by detailed remedies for specific conditions.

1.   KIDNEY CLEANSING EXERCISE

Start with the Three Regulations: steady breath, relaxed mind, Wuji posture (feet shoulder-width apart, shoulders relaxed and broad, tailbone tucked, and crown point, or top of the head, pressing up).

"Pull Down the Heavens" three times. Start with feet hip-width apart, toes pointed forward, arms relaxed by your sides. Turn palms up as you reach out and up toward the sky with both arms on the inhale. As you exhale, face the palms toward the body as you bring the hands down the center midline. As you do this, imagine white light flowing through your body and deep into the ground.

- Roll the tip of your tongue back to the soft palate on the roof of your mouth.

- Place the back of your left hand on your lower back, in the region of the right kidney.

- Bring your right arm up to the left side of your body, about eye level, palm outward.

- Inhale a blue cloud into the Kidneys as you sweep your arm to the right, gazing at the back of the right arm.

- Then exhale turbid energy as you bend forward at the waist, scooping down and across with your right arm in front of your body from right to left.

- Continue this as a circular motion. That is, inhale as you sweep your arm, at eye level, to the right, then exhale as you scoop/ sweep your arm to the left at knee level.

- Repeat this several times, then switch and do the same exercise on the left side.

- Finish by Pulling Down the Heavens three times.

2. KIDNEY HEALING SOUND

Breathe into the Kidneys and as you exhale make the *fuuu* sound out loud and then under your breath several times. You can do this in multiples of three: 3, 6, 9, . . . 36, etc. You can do this practice audibly or under your breath for five to ten minutes at a time whenever emotions of fear, fright, or shock come up for you. Focus on different events that create shock or fear.

Below is a chart listing the healing sounds for all the yin organs.

Organ	Negative Emotion	Positive Virtue	Sound
Liver	Anger, rage, frustration, resentment	Kindness	*Shuu*
Lungs	Sadness, grief	Courage	*Ssss*
Spleen	Worry, pensiveness, anxiety	Serenity, centeredness	*Huuu*
Kidneys	Fear, fright, shock	Gentleness, wisdom	*Fuuu*
Heart	Mania, overexcitation	Love, gratitude	*Haaa*

3. MICROCOSMIC ORBIT MEDITATION

The purpose of this meditation is to facilitate and reinforce the flow of Qi in the Conception and Governing Vessels, which stimulates the Central Nervous System and strengthens the spine.

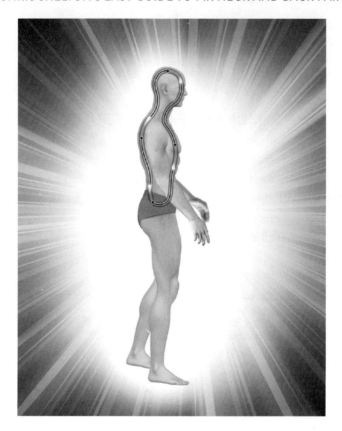

Start with the Three Regulations: steady breath, relaxed mind, Wuji posture (feet shoulder-width apart, shoulders relaxed and broad, tailbone tucked, crown point pressing up).

Place your tongue on the roof of your mouth behind your teeth. Lightly squeeze the anal sphincter muscle while relaxing your body.

As you inhale, guide Qi up the spine (the Governing Vessel) to the crown of the head. If you cannot feel the Qi, imagine it. You may imagine it as light or a color, or as blood or fluids moving upward.

As you exhale, guide Qi from the crown point down the front of the face, entering the upper palate of the mouth to the point where the tongue touches the palate.

Continuing to exhale, guide Qi down the front of the body (the Conception Vessel) to the perineum.

When Qi reaches the perineum, repeat the exercise—that is, inhale, bringing Qi up the spine, then exhale, bringing it over the crown of the head to the tongue tip and down the front to the perineum.

Repeat the exercise continuously. At the end (with your mind) bring Qi to the lower Tan Tien (an inch below the belly button in the center of the abdomen) and store it there.

4. PELVIS ALIGNMENT

Stand with feet shoulder-width apart, toes pointed forward.

Stand tall with head, shoulder, hip socket, knee, and ankle bone all in one line.

I recommend standing near a doorway to help line up the hips and shoulders.

- Place your right hand on the door jamb.

- Step forward with the left foot and land with a bent left knee.

- Keep your torso and head upright as you lunge forward, and keep the right leg straight with a locked knee.

- As you gently lunge, lift the chest and the chin slightly, looking toward the ceiling. (This will further help to elongate the plumb line.)

- Hold for about 20 seconds, then switch to the other leg.

Key Points

- Both feet need to be facing straight ahead.

- It's important to note that you should not step backward into the lunge. With the feet shoulder-width apart, step forward into the lunge.

- Walk around after you have completed the exercise.

- I've seen these three remedy strategies work miracles for my clients over the years, and they help with all the most common low back complaints.

- Get in the habit of repeating these exercises every day for maintenance and prevention.

5. CAT COW TECHNIQUE

This is an effective yet gentle technique to aid in the healing of the back. It's a great way to warm the spine and loosen everything up while stimulating the nervous system, glands, and abdominal muscles. See images on the next page.

- Start on your hands and knees with wrists directly under your shoulders and knees directly under your hips.

- Have your fingertips pointing forward and place your shins and knees hip-width apart.

- Keep your head in a centered and neutral position with a soft, unfocused gaze looking forward.

- Maintain the breath—long, steady, even, and deep, in and out through the nose.

- Start by moving into cat pose: take a breath, and as you exhale, draw your belly to your spine and round your mid-back toward the ceiling. The posture should look like a cat arching its back.

- Spread your shoulder blades apart while drawing your shoulders away from your ears.

- Point the crown of your head down toward the floor, but don't force your chin to your chest.

- Next, move into cow pose. Inhale as you drop your belly toward the ground. Lift your chin and chest, gazing up toward the ceiling.

- Inhale, coming back into cat pose. Then exhale as you return to cow pose.

- Repeat five to ten times, or whatever feels best for you.

- Stop this exercise if you feel any sharp pains in your back.

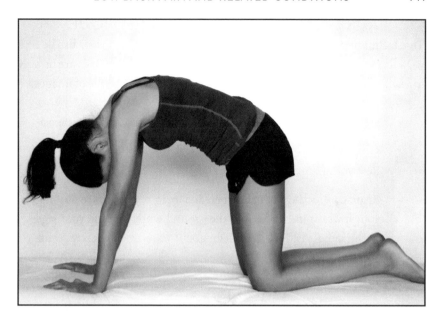

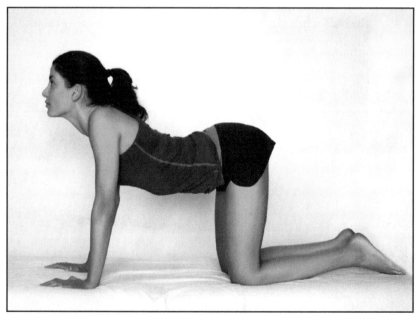

6. REVERSE CAT AND COW TECHNIQUE

This technique works best when you're lying on the floor. You can also lie on a yoga mat or massage table. Avoid lying on your bed, though. Beds are usually too soft to do this technique properly. See the following series of images.

- Start by lying on your back with your legs lifted in tabletop position, feet off the floor and the knees bent at a right angle.

- Rest your palms on your knees.

- Begin contracting your abdomen and imagine that you're pushing your lower spine down into the ground while holding your legs in the same position. Do this for about 10 seconds, then relax for about 10 seconds.

- Next, keeping your hands and legs in the same position, try to arch your back up off the floor, keeping your shoulder blades down (practitioners: you should be able to slide your hand under the back when it is arched properly). Arch for about 10 seconds. Again, rest for another 10 seconds, then repeat the process of pressing down for 10 seconds and arching for 10 seconds.

- Do this sequence five to six times, once or twice per day.

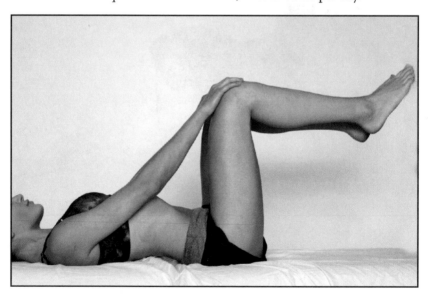

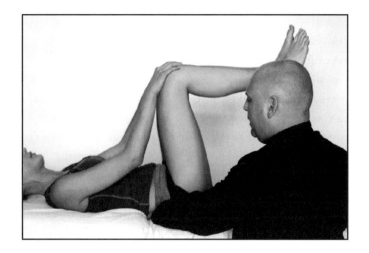

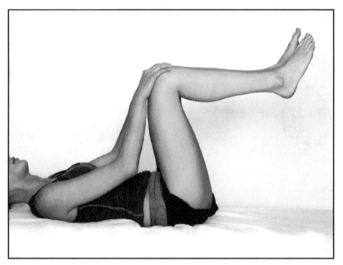

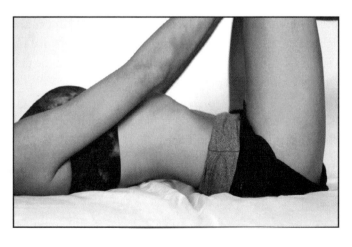

7. CHILD'S POSE

Child's pose helps relax the nervous system, stretch your back muscles, and open up your hips. See image below.

Start in a kneeling position. Drop your buttocks toward your heels and lean forward, continuing to push your buttocks down toward your heels as you reach your arms forward and rest your forehead on the floor.

Draw your arms back so they rest next to your legs, palms facing up. Inhale and exhale, slowly and deeply, for at least nine breaths.

If it's hard for you to rest your forehead on the floor, try this variation: Kneel and sit with your knees slightly apart. Lean forward, fold your arms in front of you on the floor, and rest your forehead on your arms, a pillow, or a yoga block.

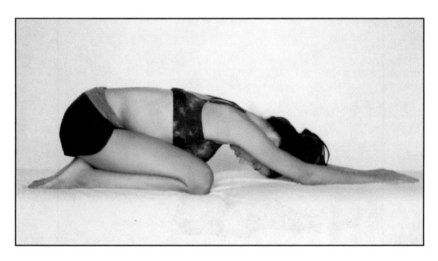

8. LUNGE STRETCH

This stretch helps align the sacroiliac (SI) joint. The SI joint connects the sacrum to the iliac bones. The sacrum is the triangular bone that runs horizontally at the base of the spine and the iliac is the brim of the pelvis. See two images on the next page.

- Kneel on one knee with the other foot forward. If you're on a hard floor, get a pillow for your knee.

- With your hands on your SI joint and fingers pointing toward the ground, inhale, lifting the chest and head. Then exhale, gliding the hips forward toward the front foot. Hold for about 15 seconds with a long, steady breath.

- Don't bounce.

- Repeat on the other side (do this just once on each side).

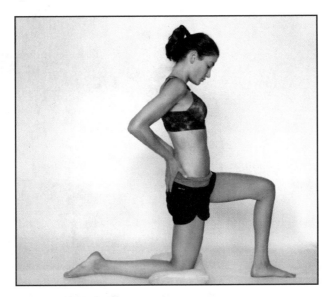

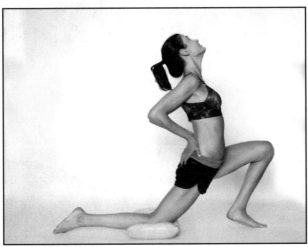

Note—this technique is extra powerful if you do the psoas stretch first.

Very important: Be sure to walk after stretching (or have your client walk) to engage the muscles.

9. TENNIS BALL PRESS/ROLL

Place two tennis balls in a long sock and push both balls all the way down to the end of the sock. (The balls should be right next to each other.) Next, tie the sock closed. Your spine will rest in the groove between the balls.

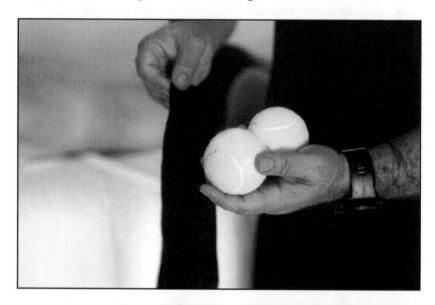

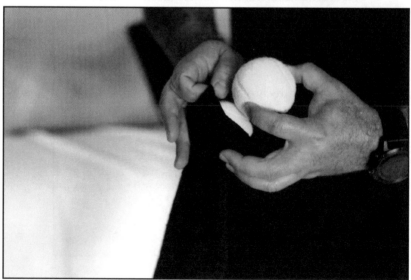

Lie on the floor or another hard surface (carpet may be too soft) with your spine between the two balls, placing them near the big bone point at the base of the neck.

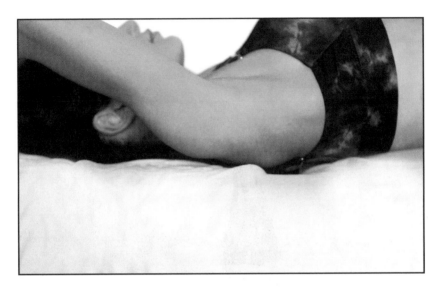

- Breathe until you feel the tension in your muscles relax. Then roll the balls down your back about half an inch to a new position and breathe until you feel those muscles relax.

- Continue relaxing the muscles and rolling down to a new position, about half an inch at a time.

- Continue this technique only until you reach the last of your free-floating ribs at the end of the rib cage.

- Important: Never position the tennis balls below the last of the free-floating ribs on your spine and never over the kidneys.

- A word of caution: If your upper or middle back is tight, this may be very uncomfortable! Try to breathe through the discomfort.

- This exercise triggers Urinary Bladder (UB) acupuncture points down the back, which in turn stimulate other points connected to various internal organs.

- This technique is especially good for hip, sciatic, and tailbone pain. Use a single tennis ball under one hip (on GB 30, UB 30, UB 34, UB 35, UB 53, and UB 54). See the following images.

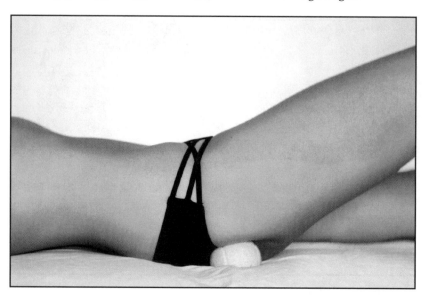

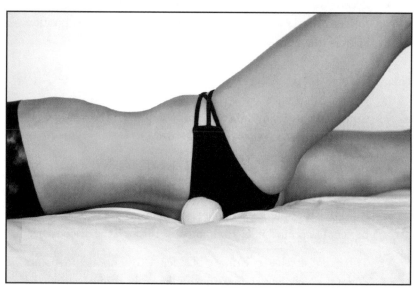

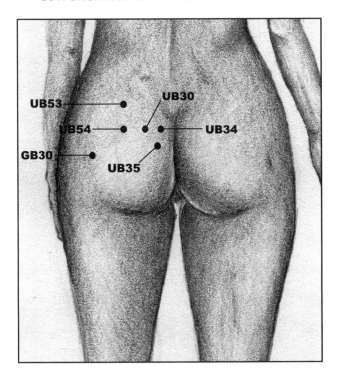

It is also beneficial to use this method for neck and shoulder issues by lying with a single tennis ball placed on SI 11, in the center of the scapula.

The tennis ball technique is a substitute for having a practitioner do deep tissue massage. Breathe through it the best you can. Also, it is important to use a tennis ball rather than a harder ball, to reduce your chance of injury.

Again, do not apply tennis balls below the rib cage. Doing so can create more back pain.

10. FOAM ROLLER TECHNIQUE

Using a foam roller on GB 32 (where your fingers rest when your arms are at your sides) will loosen up the GB channel when you're suffering from sciatica. Working this point also helps to alleviate pain in the iliotibial (IT) band (the outside of the thigh). You can place the foam roller under your glutes to help open UB 53 and UB 54. Also, rolling out the upper back is helpful for reducing tension in the lower back.

Lie on your side with the foam roller under your thigh pressing on GB 32 (or under your hip or on GB 30). See the following images.

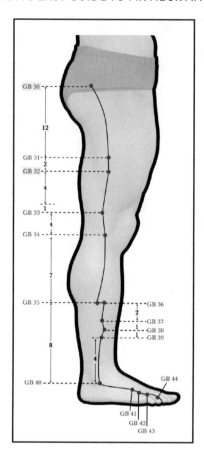

Roll up and down and side to side.

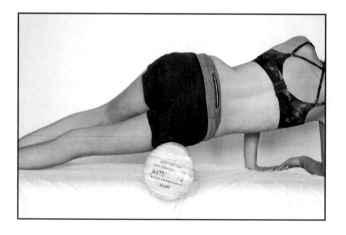

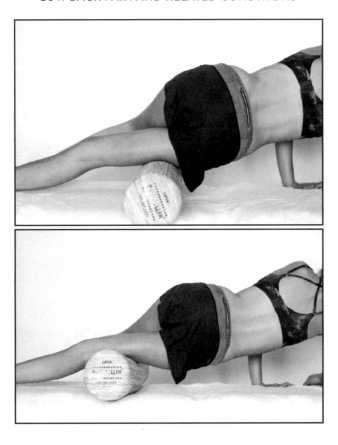

As long as it doesn't hurt your lower back, you can place the foam roller under the glutes and hips and roll back and forth.

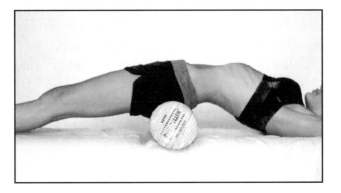

Place the foam roller under the base of the neck and upper shoulders then roll up and down to the last rib.

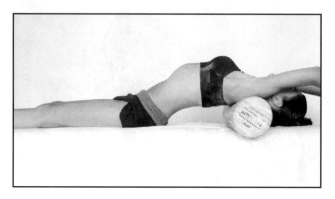

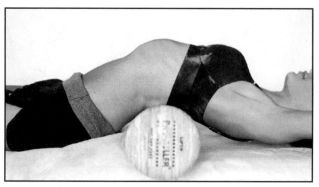

11. GUA SHA

Gua sha, also known as "coining" or "scraping," is a method of scraping the skin with a tool to release stagnant Qi, blood, and fluids in order to reduce inflammation and pain. See two images on the next page.

You'll probably need to see a practitioner for gua sha; it can be very painful to do on yourself. In fact, most people can't, because we're wired not to inflict pain on ourselves. Some report that it feels like they're being cut with a razor blade or their skin is being scraped off.

If you want to attempt it yourself, here's how:

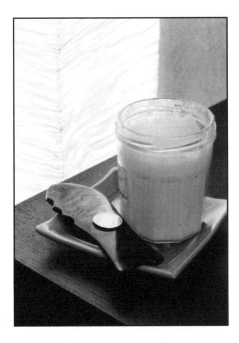

Using lots of coconut oil, rub a sterilized coin or a gua sha tool on the acupuncture channel of the legs. Rub toward the toes, not up toward the abdomen. See image below.

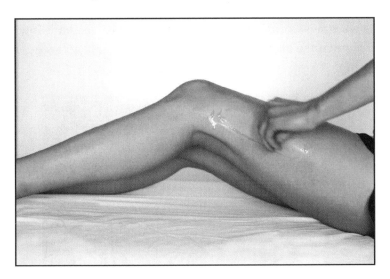

If you work up to it mentally, doing gua sha along the Liver, Gallbladder, Spleen, or other affected channels (until the area turns red or purple) will help clear blockages and allow for fresh blood and fluids to move in and heal the body.

An athlete from San Jose State University came in with a sciatic issue and I taught him how to gua sha to loosen up and alleviate nerve pain on the outside of his thigh. He did gua sha on himself every four or five days for about a month. He was able to fix the condition himself.

Warning: If you have diabetes or any other condition in which you bleed or bruise easily, this technique may be contraindicated.

12. MOXIBUSTION TECHNIQUES

Mugwort is an herb with a bit of a reputation. For centuries, the spongy plant has been ground up and burned as a way to ward off evil spirits. Today, in classical Chinese medicine, it is used in the practice of moxibustion, a blend of heat therapy and acupuncture. When mugwort is dried, the herb is called *moxa*. For this technique, moxa is burned in close proximity to the skin.

Moxibustion is painless. The herb is compressed into a stick or pole that resembles a cigar or into little balls. When lit, the moxa stick or moxa ball smolders and offers a powerful form of targeted heat therapy that's relaxing and noninvasive. Moxibustion is particularly successful in relieving chronic pain, stress, impotence, low sex drive, digestive problems, and anxiety.

As with most forms of Chinese medicine, moxibustion is intended to strengthen the blood, stimulate the flow of Qi, and enhance general well-being.

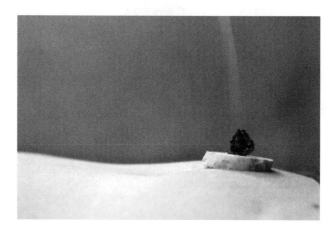

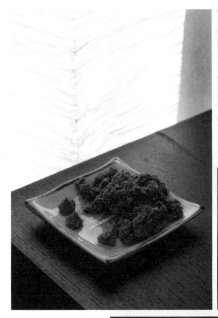
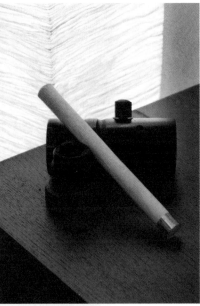
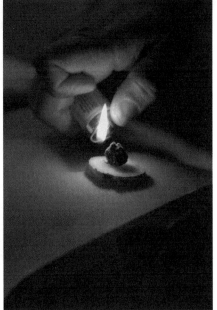

Please note: Moxibustion is sometimes contraindicated for certain diseases; therefore, please consult a licensed acupuncturist before applying this method.

Warning: Because you are dealing with a flame, you have to be careful not to start a fire or burn yourself. This technique is safer when administered by a licensed practitioner.

USING CUPPING TO RELIEVE BACK PAIN

In this section I'll introduce the basics of cupping to help you relieve your own back pain.

But first, some definitions.

You'll notice that I frequently use the term tonify. To tonify means to improve stress conditions and the overall constitution of the body. When we tonify, we build and strengthen certain organs or systems of organs. We enhance and improve the basic constitution of the body and strengthen what CCM calls your Upright Qi, or your ability to fight off external pathogens. Upright Qi is the strength of your Qi—it's the energy you are born with that comes from your parents and your environment at conception. Your Upright Qi originates in the Kidneys but is expressed through all the organs.

An example of tonifying: if your tongue is large, fat, or shows tooth marks around the edges, we know that your Spleen Qi is weak. So we tonify that organ system to improve your overall health.

Next, the various kinds of cupping.

1. CUPPING TECHNIQUES

I can hear it now. You're asking yourself, "What the heck is cupping?"

Cupping is a technique that uses a glass or plastic jar and light vacuum pressure to clear out toxins, invigorate acupuncture points, and move Qi and blood.

A cupping jar is a small round glass with a smooth rim. It is used to create a partial vacuum over the skin, which causes the blood to circulate and get pulled toward the surface of the body.

Chinese cupping dates back to the year AD 281. It was a Taoist medical practice used in the imperial courts of China. Although it is believed to have originated in China, cupping is also popular in Hong Kong, Japan, Korea,

India, and South and Central America. Thousands of years ago, animal horns were used and later, bamboo cups.

Cupping was originally practiced to remedy pulmonary diseases in conjunction with acupuncture and moxibustion. In fact, these techniques became standard remedies for chronic pulmonary diseases during the Tang Dynasty.

The cupping method is warming and promotes a free flow of Qi and blood in the meridians, dispelling cold and dampness while diminishing swelling and pain. In modern clinics, cupping is mainly used to remedy pain in the lower back, shoulders, and legs, in addition to gastrointestinal disorders such as stomachache, vomiting, and diarrhea. It is also used to remedy lung conditions, including cough and asthma. It can be used for toxic heat syndrome or for a variety of acute ailments.

There are many types of cupping techniques that result in different benefits, and some of those can only be performed by a licensed practitioner. In this chapter, I'll cover the few that can be done safely at home.

Traditionally, acupuncturists use what is referred to as fire cupping. This technique involves soaking a piece of a cotton ball in rubbing alcohol, holding it with a pair of forceps, and lighting it on fire. The lit cotton ball is placed into a glass jar (see images below). The flame sucks out all the oxygen in the jar, creating a vacuum. The jar is then turned over and placed on a particular part of the body. Because of the safety hazard involved with using fire, I recommend that you avoid these and instead use the suction cupping sets.

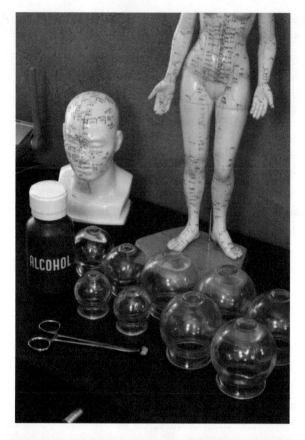

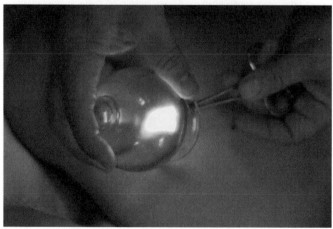

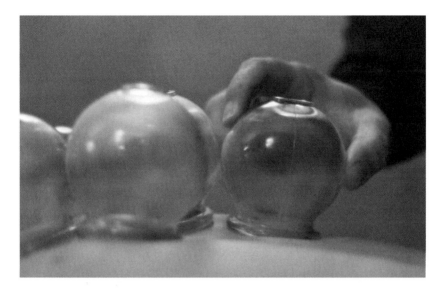

Warning: As with all other techniques recommended in this book, you are advised to consult your primary health care provider to make sure this is safe for you or your loved ones. There may be contraindications with certain types of medical conditions and/or medications.

There are some acupuncture points that are contraindicated for cupping. For example, it's not recommended that you cup over the abdominal region (where soft organs are), on the heart, or over the kidneys on the lower back.

The maximum amount of cupping time should be no more than 15 minutes for healthy adults. With children, the elderly, or anyone with a febrile disease or hampered constitution, cup for seven to eight minutes only.

I recommend placing the cups only on acupuncture points listed in this section to help with various conditions affecting the lower back, middle back, and neck, or for shoulder pain. For weak cupping, only one to two pumps are recommended. For medium cupping, three pumps, and for strong cupping, four to five pumps maximum.

2. FOUR TYPES OF CUPPING
You'll notice cupping referred to by its strength. Here's what that means:

2.1. Weak Cupping
Weak suction is effective for excess heat conditions such as stress and stomach problems or for neurological conditions including paralysis and post-stroke

weakness. According to Chinese medicine, this method is intended to remove stagnation while tonifying weak Qi and blood without depleting the energy of people who are weak or frail.

The suction used in this method is less strong, and therefore, so is the intensity, making it a gentle remedy that can be used on people of any age.

Weak cupping uses only one or two pumps.

2.2. Medium Cupping

The suction used in medium cupping is firmer than with weak cupping and can be safely administered to children over the age of seven, as well as adults.

Medium cupping is indicated for muscular pains, stress-related conditions, and children's ailments. If you use cupping on kids aged seven to twelve, back off if they feel discomfort. Teens can usually tolerate more because their constitutions can handle it.

Use three pumps for medium cupping.

2.3. Strong Cupping

The suction in this method is the firmest, with four to five pumps, and therefore can drain energy from the person.

Because strong cupping manipulates significant amounts of blood and Qi, it often leaves marks on the body.

The purpose of strong cupping is to improve blood circulation and remove pathogens that cause diseases. This method also helps with painful or swollen joints, low and mid-back pain, and frozen shoulder syndrome.

2.4. Moving Cupping

This style should be done only by a skilled licensed practitioner. Moving cupping applies strong therapy to a larger area of the body, usually on the Urinary Bladder channel on the back.

The practitioner applies generous amounts of coconut or another massage oil to the back over the whole surface area, especially the ribs and shoulders. A single cup is placed on the back, and because of the lubrication, the practitioner can slide the cup along, encompassing all the acupuncture points there.

Moving cupping is effective for excess heat conditions of the skin such as acne, skin lesions, and inflammation. It also benefits neurological conditions like paralysis and post-stroke weakness, as well as painful, swollen joints, by manipulating excess energy and bringing the heat to the surface of the skin.

I normally recommend not moving the cup below the free-floating ribs of the back. Also, do not do this technique over the kidneys or in the kidney region.

Let's look at acupressure techniques next.

ACUPRESSURE TO RELIEVE BACK PAIN

There are a couple of acupressure methods I recommend when you're suffering from back pain. Both are things you should do immediately because they will reinforce the psoas stretch.

Let's start with two of the most common acupressure techniques.

FOOT REFLEXOLOGY

Foot reflexology is an ancient art originally practiced by the early Egyptians. It's a form of acupressure, but it's also a science of its own.

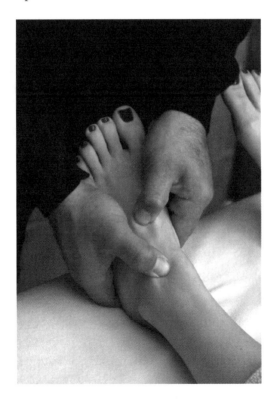

Foot reflexology is based on the theory that areas of the feet are composed of zones and reflex points that correspond to your glands, organs, and bodily systems. During reflexology, pressure is applied to these areas using thumb, finger, and hand methods. One of its main benefits is reducing stress. Reflexology can indirectly help people regain balance and restore proper functionality of the internal organs. Foot reflexology and massage promote physiological improvements and restore the natural balance of the body while revitalizing the organs and related systems.

In regard to relieving back pain, reflexology is used to gently dredge and clear certain acupuncture points and meridians on the feet and toes. (Dredging is a technique used in acupressure in which you apply pressure to a specific point, massage firmly, and imagine the pain as a dark cloud leaving the channel.) In addition, reflexology is combined with other techniques to help harmonize the internal organs that contribute to particular dysfunctions.

Reflexology is valuable in locating high-stress or high-tension areas in the body and can be used to encourage natural healing. Since 85 percent of all health problems are linked to stress and negative emotions, reflexology greatly aids in healing. It is always better if you can have someone help you with this technique—and of course, nothing feels better than having somebody massage your feet! But you can still apply pressure to the different areas by yourself and get the same results.

The chart above shows what areas of the body you're stimulating as you massage or perform reflexology. If you add the acupressure points on your feet, you're taking it a step further.

Your goal? Pay attention to the chart, massage certain areas, and be aware of your emotional state or what comes up emotionally as you work. Also, notice what organs you're stimulating. Then refer to the section on the acupuncture points at the end of this chapter. Read that section and begin to understand—what does LV 3 do? Why am I pressing or massaging this place on my foot?

For example, if you massage the top of your foot and feel something like small sand particles, beads, or pebbles underneath the skin, you may be having feelings of being unloved or unwanted. In CCM, that's the stomach meridian, but in reflexology, that area represents the chest. Combining reflexology with acupressure helps you acknowledge these feelings. At the same time, you're stimulating and helping to strengthen the Stomach and Spleen. So you can use the information you learn both ways. I call it reflexology with a twist.

Get familiar with the reflexology chart but also the location of acupuncture points. Reinforce your body's self-curative abilities by noticing the organs that work together.

For example, if you massage LV 3 or GB 43, you should also rub or gently pull the top of the foot near the toes and project the Qi out the toe. Clear the LV and GB meridians to reinforce the exercise. Over the years, I've found that working this way has the greatest benefit.

ACUPRESSURE

Acupressure is an ancient Chinese healing method that involves applying pressure to certain acupuncture meridian points, not only to relieve pain but to facilitate the healing process of various diseases, pain, inflammation, and neurological issues.

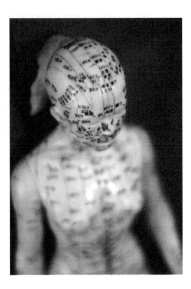

The body has twelve "regular" acupuncture meridians that feed into what is referred to as the twelve regular organs. These acupuncture meridians start, and in many cases end, in the fingertips and toes. If not there, they end and begin on the torso and face.

There are also eight "extraordinary" meridians that connect the left and right sides of the body, the front and back, and the upper and lower torso. These influence the function of the extraordinary organs—the testes, ovaries, and brain.

In acupressure, we use the same acupuncture points that acupuncturists use, except with firm pressure of the hands rather than a needle. The fingers press or massage key acupuncture points to stimulate your body's self-curative abilities.

As you press these points, you release muscular tension and promote the circulation of blood, lymph fluid, and Qi. You can apply acupressure to yourself or have it applied by a certified or licensed practitioner. You can also imagine tonifying by placing your mind's intent on projecting Qi into a point as you rub or massage it.

An acupuncturist can sedate, reduce, or tonify by the way they insert, angle, and turn the needle. You can also sedate, reduce, or tonify with acupressure and Qigong but with your intention and mind focus rather than a needle.

EXAMPLES: COMBINING QIGONG, CUPPING, AND ACUPRESSURE

As I mentioned at the start of this section, all these healing strategies complement and build on each other.

Before you try this yourself, reread the cupping warning in the above section.

The following methods indirectly reinforce the number one and number two primary techniques in healing back pain.

1. Order a suction cupping set

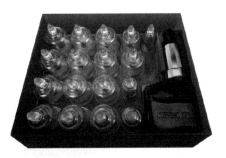

2. Do three or four pumps on LV 13 and LV 14.

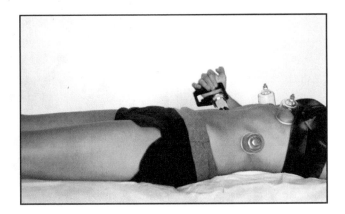

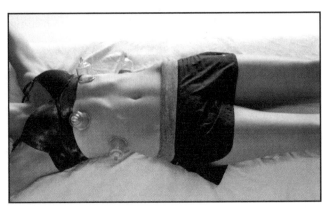

3. Lie back and relax for 10 or 15 minutes, depending on your age group and circumstances mentioned in the cupping section.

4. Once you're done, remove the cups.

5. Using acupressure, massage and dredge (apply pressure, massage firmly, and imagine the pain as a dark cloud leaving the channel) LV 3 between your toes. See images below.

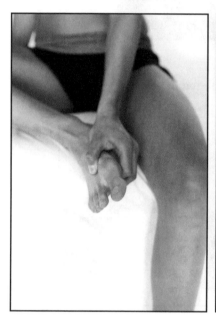 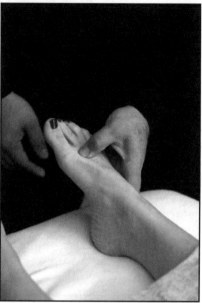

6. Finally, practice the Qigong techniques to reinforce healing.

You can do acupressure in the context of Qigong to see greater healing benefits. Press on a point and project your Qi—with your mind's intent—while massaging the point. It's not just about remedying the specific area of the lower back, but auxiliary points as well.

Remember that your Liver plays a major role in back pain. Cup LV 14 and imagine a line that runs straight down from the nipple to the sixth intercostal space between the ribs. After that, I recommend that you massage and do acupressure on LV 3 between your big toe and second toe. When you use acupressure this way, you're projecting Qi into the point to either sedate or tonify.

To distinguish between cupping and acupressure, think of it this way: acupressure involves massaging and focusing intention on a point, whereas cupping groups multiple points to increase the communication between them. It enhances their influence on the organs and the internal/external environment. It uses suction to increase the movement of blood and fluids as well as Qi.

For example, LV 13 is a direct acupuncture point for the Liver, but you can also use it to reduce emotions related to anger.

All these remedies will help relieve immediate pain. Now let's look at how you can prevent that pain from returning in the future.

LOW BACK PAIN MAINTENANCE AND PREVENTION

Here you'll learn lifestyle changes that will help you become stronger and healthier. Note that all these techniques complement and build on each other. You don't need to choose one or another. Start with what makes the most sense for you and add other healing modalities as you are able. You'll notice improvements within a short time, but your health will improve greatly in the long run.

First, we'll look at the physical practices.

1. QIGONG FOR BACK PAIN

If you want to heal your back pain, I can't recommend Qigong or Tai Chi highly enough.

I like to say that Qigong involves simple practices that create profound results. It will help you improve your posture, breath, and focus.

Below are some of the most helpful Qigong practices for lower back pain:

- Microcosmic orbit meditation
- Brushing the meridians
- Massaging the yang organs
- Kidney cleansing exercise
- Kidney healing sound (*fuuu*)
- Heart cleansing exercise
- Heart healing sound (*haaa*)
- White pearl meditation

- Liver cleansing exercise
- Liver healing sound (*shuu*)
- Spleen cleansing exercise
- Spleen healing sound (*huuu*)

Detailed instructions on these are included in the DIY remedy sections of chapters 9 and 10. Check out those chapters to get started.

Deep breathing practices like the white pearl meditation are extremely useful in balancing your internal emotional well-being and strengthening your back. The white pearl meditation helps you deal with fear, which is one of the major contributors to low back pain.

I recommend that you do all the basic Qigong five-organ cleansing exercises (that can be found in this book or on my YouTube channel) for the Liver, Heart, Spleen, Lung, and Kidneys every day for balance and then come back to concentrate on the specific movements in this list a bit more. If you don't have time for a full session or if you're feeling lazy, you can concentrate on the Liver and Kidney moves.

Please visit our YouTube channel, @chrissheltonqigong, and the playlist "30 Days of Qigong to Better Health" for a full list of Qigong videos you can follow along with.

2. TAI CHI FOR BACK PAIN

Tai Chi is another great practice that gently strengthens your muscles as well as your tendons and ligaments. It's an excellent way to improve focus, straighten your lower back, increase flexibility, decrease anxiety and hypertension, increase your overall consciousness, and increase energy. Compared to Qigong, Tai Chi is more physical. It benefits a greater amount of your body overall, but the movements are more complex and it takes longer to learn.

According to studies conducted at Stanford and Harvard, Tai Chi has been proven to help with high blood pressure. That's because it requires you to stay focused in the present moment. The waxing and waning movements of the legs increase blood and lymph flow, which helps strengthen the immune system and our ability to fight off disease.

We also have Tai Chi videos on our @chrissheltonqigong YouTube channel. Check them out and subscribe to see our latest.

FOOD REMEDIES FOR LOW BACK PAIN

As a lifestyle change, you'll want to start thinking of using food as medicine and not just fuel.

Chinese medicine is useful for helping diagnose health imbalances, especially illnesses, and even chronic pain. The misconception that the food you eat doesn't contribute to low back pain, or back, neck, and shoulder pain in general, is just that—a misconception. A fallacy.

According to Chinese nutrition, a healthy, vibrant body requires a whole-foods program. That's because your diet plays a vital role in your health balance. Being aware of the properties of the foods you eat, including what organs and organ systems they affect and how, can help you tailor your diet to alleviate symptoms of illness.

In general, your meals should consist of lightly cooked or blanched vegetables. Blanched means that you sauté, bake, boil, or steam your vegetables for no longer than two or three minutes. Any leafy green vegetable will turn bright green when it has been blanched for about three minutes.

Vegetables should make up between 40 percent and 60 percent of your diet. Complex carbohydrates should make up about 30 percent, and lean, high-quality protein should make up about 10 percent. That means when you look at your plate, half should be vegetables, a little more than one-fourth healthy carbs, and a small portion, protein.

Ideally, your diet should consist of fragrant, lightly spiced meals with blanched vegetables and healthy fats like avocado, coconut, fish oil, and ghee.

The type of protein matters. For example, if you're aiming to build your Kidneys, the 10 percent of your diet that's protein should come from fish. If you're more interested in building your blood, that 10 percent should come from red meat.

Make sure that all your protein comes from high-quality sources, meaning it should be unprocessed, organic, and grass fed as much as possible.

If you suspect that your back problems are due to resentment or old anger, some of the vegetables and foods that will help are basil, ginger, mustard greens, brussels sprouts, lemon, mint, basil, and small amounts of pickled vegetables. Some liquids that will help include soy sauce, apple cider vinegar, and small amounts of coffee.

If you feel, from reading the descriptions in the previous chapter, that your low back pain is due to a Kidney deficiency, then foods like black beans, adzuki beans, tofu, Bosc pears, tangerines, apricots, peaches, pork, small packages of seaweed snacks, and smaller saltwater fish like sardines will benefit you, as well as cooking with kelp granules.

Avoid excessive amounts of alcohol; caffeine; white flour; greasy, fatty, or fried foods; and sugar. Consume minimal dairy and eggs. Try to avoid fluoridated water, artificial colors and flavors, artificial preservatives, and meat pumped with antibiotics.

Mealtimes should be stress free. This means no heated conversations at the dinner table, no eating in front of the TV, and no arguing while eating. Avoid eating on the run, standing while eating, not being mindful while eating, or eating too quickly.

All these minor adjustments add up and will contribute to balancing out discord in your digestive system and the function of your internal organs, which will contribute to decreasing the stress that causes back problems.

Finally, see the Location and Function of Acupoints to Relieve Back Pain guide on the resources page at http://chrissheltonseasyguide.com or scan the QR code for information on all the acupuncture points referenced in this chapter.

REMEDIES FOR COMMON LOW BACK CONDITIONS

The following is a list of the most common lower back conditions and the areas of extremities that are subsequently affected.

As you will see, the root cause of most of these conditions is the same. Symptoms manifest differently depending on the location of the problem and which nerves it's affecting.

Before we go further, I must be firm in saying that if you have any type of low back pain that is escalating and/or numbness of the extremities for more than a few days, see your doctor.

Why? Most of the time, back pain, sciatica, tailbone pain, bulging disks, and lumbar stenosis aren't life-threatening. However, these conditions can sometimes be a sign of an injury that you're unaware of, or in rare cases, cancer. You can get an MRI scan or an X-ray to look for signs of injury or disease, such as a bone fracture, tumor, or cancer pressing on the bone and/ or nerves.

Even if you've had one or more spinal injections or have had surgery for back pain, hip pain, sciatica, or lumbar stenosis—and despite all you've done, you are still experiencing pain—the following strategies can help relieve your symptoms and get you back to enjoying the quality of life that you deserve.

Read the descriptions of the conditions that concern you. Apply the recommended remedy protocols. You'll find detailed explanations of each technique in the "DIY Remedies" section below.

1. GENERAL LOW BACK PAIN

Most people experience mild to moderate low back pain by the age of 35. Sometimes it can be due to sitting for too long, not getting enough sleep, lifting something the wrong way, being overweight, not exercising, or having tight muscles in general.

Regardless of your pain level, the problem usually originates somewhere else in the body unless your back is directly injured (e.g., car accident, surgery).

In almost all cases, the problem is the psoas muscle deep in the abdomen as well as the Kidneys and/or Liver being out of balance. These have been the root causes of all the various types of back conditions I've seen in my 20 years of clinical practice.

Emotions like fear, fright, or shock as well as aging, too much sexual release, overwork, and excessive alcohol intake deplete the Kidneys. Anger, old anger, and resentment impact the Liver and Gallbladder and have the same effect.

Lower back problems are more common in women than in men because of Kidney depletion. Remember from the previous chapter that for women, back problems are harder to fix if they are holding on to resentment toward a male figure. In these cases, the issue would be the Liver rather than the Kidneys and would include PTSD from a traumatic event—any type of abuse, especially molestation or rape.

If you've been in a car accident or have had a fall or other injury to the spine, the following techniques can still be used for a speedy recovery.

Your whole body is connected through fascia, the connective tissue that holds everything together. Tensegrity, the principle used in building suspension bridges, applies to the human body as well; what happens to one part of the body will affect another.

The shoulders and back usually trigger each other, so you must loosen up your shoulders to reinforce any work done to release the lower back. There is a similar cross-pattern between the hips and shoulders. What happens at the left hip can affect the right shoulder and vice versa.

So be sure to read chapter 10 on neck and shoulder issues.

On the following pages is a list of techniques to alleviate back pain, along with page numbers, to easily find specific techniques.

See DIY Remedies (starting with top three remedies, pages 130–35): Demonstration of reverse cat and cow (142–43), cat and cow (140–41), child's pose (144), and foam roller on glutes, hips, and upper back (149–52). Lie on tennis balls UB 13 to UB 21 (146–49). Tai Chi, Qigong: especially Kidney, Liver, Heart healing sound, and cleansing exercises (167–68). Cup LV 13, LV 14 (165); a few days later, ST 19, ST 20, and CV 15 (173–74). Repeat when marks are gone. Dredge LV 2, LV 3, GB 41, GB 42, and GB 43 (166, 173, 174, 176).

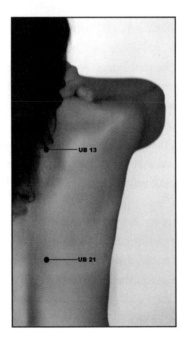

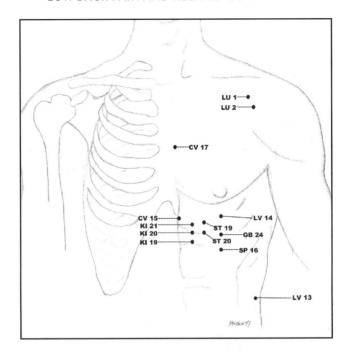

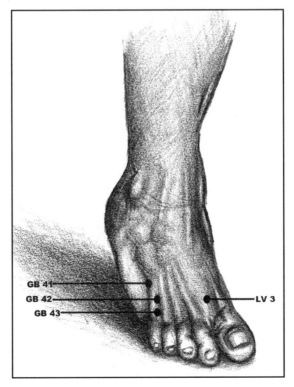

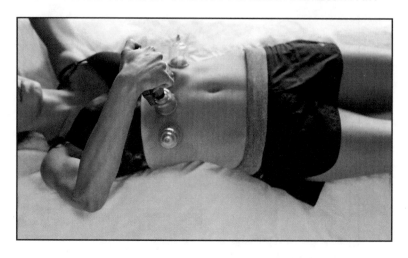

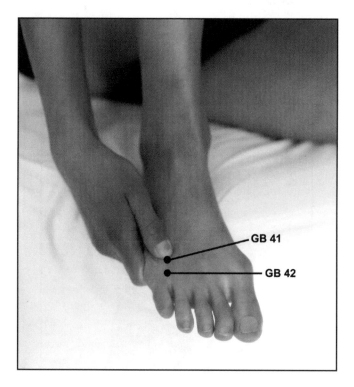

2. LUMBAR STENOSIS

A stenosis occurs any time an opening closes or constricts. For example, if you had a stenosis of the artery walls in the heart, it would mean that your artery was blocked.

When it comes to back pain, stenosis is the result of compressed discs of the vertebrae. This compression causes a closing of the spinal canal, affecting the nerves that flow out from the spinal canal and feed into the extremities, organs, and all the parts of the body.

The root cause of this compression is the psoas muscle. This huge muscle originates in the groin, attaches to the femur bone, wraps around the hip and goes around the lower lumbar region and all the way up the thoracic spine.

The psoas keeps the spine erect. If it is too tight on one side or the other of the spine, this will cause the spinal canal to close, creating stenosis and pinching of the nerves.

Unfortunately, if you decide to have surgery or spinal injections without addressing the psoas, those procedures may help temporarily but the condition will show up somewhere else on the spine because the root cause (a tight psoas) wasn't addressed.

See DIY Remedies (starting with top three remedies, pages 130–35): Top three, reverse cat and cow (142–43), cat and cow (140–41), tennis ball press on UB 30, UB 34, UB 35, UB 54, and GB 30 (147–49). Lunge stretch (144–45). Foam roller on glutes, hips, and upper back (149–52). Gua sha in a downward motion on GB 31, GB 32, and GB 33 on the affected leg (153). Do this once or twice a week until pain subsides. Gua sha on any points of the leg that are numb or tender. Do child's pose (144). Place cups on GB 32 and GB 33 for 10–15 minutes (see image on 176). Do this once or twice within a one-month period. If there are still cupping marks from previous sessions, don't place cups over those same areas; place them either above or below the previous points. Practice Tai Chi and Qigong, especially the Kidney, Liver, Heart healing sound and cleansing exercises. Cup LV 13 and LV 14 (see image on next page and on 165); a few days later, ST 19 and ST 20, then KI 20, KI 21, CV 15, GB 24, and SP 16 (173–74). Repeat when marks are gone. Dredge LV 2, LV 3, and GB 43 (166, 173).

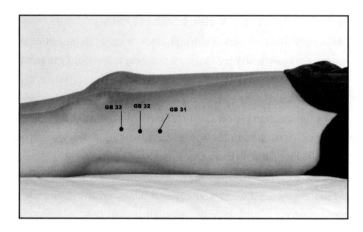

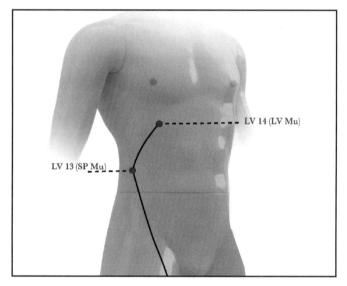

3. BULGING, HERNIATED, OR RUPTURED DISCS

Once again, each of these conditions is caused by a tight psoas muscle. The differentiating factor is the severity of trauma to the disc and the nerves.

A bulging disc is a common occurrence that results when a vertebra presses against an adjacent disc. The disc is essentially pushed out of its normal place and starts impinging on nearby spinal nerves, causing great discomfort. This condition can be extremely painful. A herniated disc, also referred to as a slipped or ruptured disc, occurs when the soft jelly-like center of the disc, or its nucleus, breaks through a tear in the tough, rubbery exterior, known as the annulus.

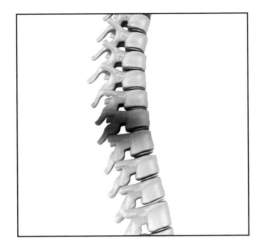

See DIY Remedies (starting with top three remedies, pages 130–35): Top three, reverse cat and cow (142–43), cat and cow (140–41), tennis ball press on UB 30, UB 34, UB 35, UB 54, and GB 30 (147–49). Child's pose (144), Tai Chi, Qigong (especially the Kidney, Liver, Heart healing sound and cleansing exercises). Cup LV 13 and LV 14 and a few days later ST 19, ST 20, and CV 15 (165, 173); repeat when marks are gone. Then KI 20, KI 21, CV 15, GB 24, and SP 16 (173–74). Repeat when marks are gone. Dredge LV 2, LV 3, and GB 43 (166, 174, 199). Foam roller on glutes, hips, and upper back (150–52).

4. SCIATICA

Sciatica affects more than three million people a year in the United States and is more commonly seen in men. It generally affects those 18 to 50.

Sciatica develops when tension in the lower back pinches the longest nerve in the body—the sciatic nerve. This nerve runs from the lower back to the hips and buttocks, then down the outside of each leg.

Sciatic nerve pain can be felt along the thigh, through the buttocks, and anywhere in the leg or foot (even toes). Many times my clients will feel a burning sensation that starts running down the outside of one of the legs. Then the pain seems to disappear for a while but shows up later in the foot or toes. The two major complaints with sciatica are burning and numbness.

Sciatica doesn't show up unannounced. There are always conditions preceding it, and usually those signs have been ignored. In other words, if or when you see the initial warning signs, take them seriously.

You may have experienced groin pain or lower back stiffness/tightness and thought it was just something you had to put up with. It's not your fault. Most people—even some doctors—don't know how to address these early warning signs.

Sciatica is caused by a herniated, bulging, or ruptured disc; a bone spur on the spine; or spinal stenosis. If you're experiencing low back or groin pain, it's a sign that one of your vertebrae is compressing a disk and starting to pinch a nerve. The longer that pinching goes on, the more irritated your sciatic nerve will get. Next thing you know, you'll have sciatica.

Tai Chi is particularly beneficial for sciatica because the legs are used so much during Tai Chi practice. The posture called Wuji elongates the lumbar spine by tucking the sacrum, helping alleviate pressure on the sciatic nerve.

I have suffered from sciatic nerve pain a few times. Once was when I was into heavy weightlifting. I was doing a seated shoulder press with two 85-pound dumbbells. I bent down to pick up the weights and felt a pull in my SI joint. I ignored the pain, telling myself, "Don't be a wimp!" I finished the set.

A few days later, I had a difficult car ride due to hip pain and a rough night sleeping on the floor (thinking that would remedy the situation). However, early the next morning when I tried to sit up, I actually felt the cartilage tear in my hip. It was the worst pain ever. That tear shifted all those vertebrae and cut off the nerves to my feet. I felt a burning pain down the outside of my leg. It disappeared at the knee and then showed up again in my big toe. It was so painful, it felt like the bone was trying to push through the skin of my big toe.

Tai Chi benefits sciatica in particular because it provides a gentle stretching and strengthening of the legs and hips and because of the previously mentioned tucking of the sacrum. It helps you develop better body mechanics and alignment, which in turn alleviates pressure on the lower lumbar, which then takes pressure off the nerves—specifically the sciatic nerve that comes down from the lower lumbar to your feet and toes.

See DIY Remedies (starting with top three remedies, pages 130–35): Top three, Tai Chi, Qigong (especially the Kidney, Liver, Heart healing sound and cleansing exercises), gua sha on GB 31 to GB 33 (152–53), and lunge stretch (144–45). Foam roller on glutes, hips, and upper back. Foam roller on outside of leg on GB 31 and GB 32 (149–51). Magnetic therapy using small magnets on UB 30, UB 34, UB 35, UB 53, and UB 54 (149, also good for sacrum and tailbone pain). Reverse cat and cow (142–43), cat and cow (140–41), child's pose (144). Cup LV 13 and LV 14 and a few days later ST 19 and ST 20 (165, 176); repeat when marks are gone. Then cup GB 24, SP 16, CV 15, KI 20, and KI 21 (173–74).

Especially for sciatica: Gua sha the GB meridian on the outside of the leg, following the sciatic nerve down the length of the leg (150–51). Do this about once a week. Also use this technique if you have knee pain or pain radiating into your shins. If you're a practitioner, the gua sha points are GB 31 to GB 33 (176), UB 40, and KI 10 (see leg images below). Cup UB 34, UB 35, and GB 30 (148–49). Do this once or twice within a month. If there still are cupping marks from a previous session, don't place cups over those same areas; place them either above or below the previous points.

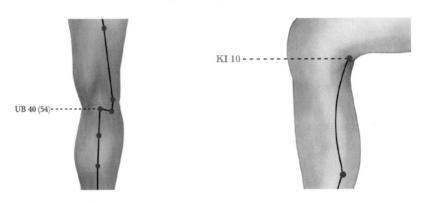

5. SACRUM AND TAILBONE PAIN

The tailbone is technically called the *coccyx*. Depending on the severity of pain and how long it's been there, you may have been diagnosed with a condition called coccydynia.

Pregnant women sometimes get tailbone pain during the last trimester of pregnancy, when ligaments that connect to the tailbone loosen to make room for the baby. Coccyx pain is often related to a fall or injury as well. It can occur from sitting too long or as the result of the psoas muscle being too tight. On rare occasions, there can be a tumor or cancer attached to the bone. The following suggestions are useful for all conditions with sacrum, coccyx, or tailbone pain.

See DIY Remedies (starting with top three remedies, pages 130–35): Top three, reverse cat and cow (142–43), cat and cow (140–41), lunge stretch (144–45), tennis ball press on UB 30, UB 34, UB 35, UB 53, UB 54, and

GB 30 (146, 148–49). Foam roller on glutes, hips, and upper back (150–52). Magnet therapy applied with surgical tape along GV 3 of the spine, on the lower back, and on UB 30, UB 34, UB 35, UB 53, UB 54, and GB 30 (149). You can order small magnets, and take surgical tape and place them over the Urinary Bladder points listed above. For more information about magnet therapy, refer to the glossary. Cup on UB 30, UB 34, UB 54, and GB 30 (149). Then KI 20, KI 21, CV 15, GB 24, and SP 16 (173). Repeat when marks are gone. Do this once or twice in a one-month period. If there still are cupping marks from previous sessions, don't place cups over those same areas; place them lateral to the previous points.

6. SI JOINT PAIN

SI joint pain is technically called sacroiliac pain, aka butt pain. The sacroiliac joints connect the sacrum to the right and left iliac bones and are made up of cartilage.

If you were to lift up your shirt, pull your pants down a little, and look at your backside in a mirror, you'd see the small dimples at the base of your lower back that correspond with the location of the SI joints. This area is called the posterior superior iliac spine (PSIS).

The sacrum is a triangular bone in the lower part of the spine, centrally located below the lumbar spine. At the tip of the sacrum is your coccyx.

Sacroiliac pain is a dysfunction of the lower back. You may notice pain toward the top of the buttocks on the left and/or right side of the spine. This pain can radiate to the groin, hips, back of the thighs, and feet. Many clients notice that standing for long periods of time or climbing stairs can aggravate it.

Sacroiliac joint dysfunction is a contributing factor in 15 percent to 30 percent of people with persistent low back pain. Again, the psoas muscle is the main contributor, but other muscles of the buttocks are involved as well, including the gluteus maximus, the gluteus medius, and the thoracolumbar fascia (the connective tissue between the middle back and lower back).

Besides the techniques mentioned above, the following are useful to help alleviate inflammation and symptoms so you can fix the condition.

See DIY Remedies (starting with top three remedies, pages 130–35): Top three, reverse cat and cow (142–43), cat and cow (140–41), lunge stretch (144–45), tennis ball press on UB 30, UB 34, UB 35, UB 53, UB 54, and GB 30 (146, 148–49). Foam roller on glutes, hips, and upper back (149–52). Magnet therapy applied with surgical tape along GV 3 of the spine, on the lower back, and on UB 30, UB 34, UB 35, UB 53, UB 54, and GB 30. You can order small magnets, and take surgical tape and place them over the Urinary Bladder points listed above. For more information about magnet therapy, refer to the glossary. Cup on UB 30, UB 34, UB 54, and GB 30. Then KI 20, KI 21, CV 15, GB 24, and SP 16 (149, 173). Repeat when marks are gone. Do this once or twice in a one-month period. If there still are cupping marks from previous sessions, don't place cups over those same areas; place them lateral to the previous points.

7. SCOLIOSIS

This condition affects babies, kids, teens, and adults. It refers to a sideways curvature of the spine that occurs most often during a growth spurt or just before puberty.

The type of scoliosis referred to in this section is not congenital scoliosis, which begins in the womb as the baby's back is developing, nor is it a condition like cerebral palsy or muscular dystrophy. If you're an adult or in your late teens and have recently received a diagnosis of scoliosis, understanding how the psoas functions can help you comprehend how it can show up at this time in your life.

See DIY Remedies (starting with top three remedies, pages 130–35): Top three, reverse cat and cow (142–43), cat and cow (140–41), lunge stretch (144–45), tennis ball press on UB 30, UB 34, UB 35, UB 53, UB 54, and GB 30 (146, 148–49); also UB 41 to UB 45 on the upper back between the shoulder blades (see images immediately below). Foam roller on glutes, hips, and upper back (149–52).

8. DROP-LEG SYNDROME AND ATROPHY

This syndrome is also called foot drop or drop foot and is a general term for when someone has difficulty lifting their legs as they walk. As a result, the front part of the foot drags or drops on the ground.

This condition occurs when the nerves exiting the lower back and sacrum (the fibular nerve and the sciatic nerve that extends into the lower part of the legs and feet) become malnourished due to an impingement in the lower lumbar and sacral area. This weakens the communication between the back and the feet, causing a neurological and muscular deficiency. This condition

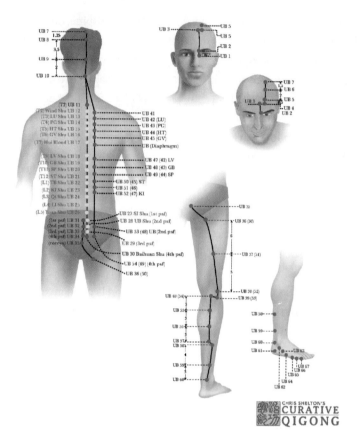

is symptomatic of a bigger problem in the lower lumbar region that has not been addressed effectively.

Sometimes this condition is only temporary, but if it continues long term, the person will suffer from atrophy of the lower leg or legs. Atrophy is a decrease in size, or a wasting away, of the muscle mass, cells, and tissues— in this case due to poor nourishment resulting from the loss of the nerves' supply.

Unfortunately, drop-leg syndrome is usually treated with medication and surgeries, with no guarantee of a positive outcome. In my experience and clinical practice, this condition is reversible. However, if the degeneration of the muscle and nerves is so severe that the atrophy is quite prevalent, the person needs to see a qualified CCM practitioner to help increase blood and nerve flow down to the feet. You can still help yourself by doing the DIY remedies plus gua sha along the Gallbladder and Liver meridians on the inside and outside of the leg and into the shin and calf.

The following remedies are recommended if you have this condition or if you're a practitioner helping someone with drop-leg syndrome.

See DIY Remedies (starting with top three remedies, pages 130–35): Top three, gua sha on the outside of the calf and thigh muscle to stimulate the sciatic nerve and the Gallbladder meridian (149). Do this once a week. Gua sha on LV 9 down to LV 8 (see image of thigh and leg below). Foam roller on glutes (150–52), hips, and upper back (150–51, 182). Foam roller on outside of leg on GB 31 and GB 32 (150–51, 176). Lunge stretch (144–45), cat and cow (140–41), reverse cat and cow (142–43), child's pose (144). Cup on GB 32 and GB 33 (176). Dredge LV 3, GB 43 (173), and cup LV 13 and LV 14; a few days later ST 19 and ST 20, then KI 20, KI 21, CV 15, GB 24, and SP 16 (173–76). Repeat when marks are gone.

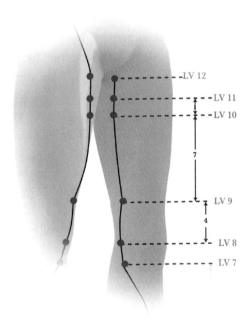

9. HIP OR GROIN PAIN

Unless you have torn or pulled your groin playing sports or slipped on something and landed the wrong way, most groin pain is a precursor to your back going out. Your body is always giving you warning signs, and hip or groin pain is one of them. Listening to those warning signs and understanding what they mean in order to help prevent disease is the foundation of Chinese medicine and Qigong.

My clients often tell me they notice groin pain when they sit for long periods or while they're walking. They try to stand up and feel a pulling sensation in the groin, hear a clicking sensation, or feel as though their groin gets stuck as they move to stand. Groin pain is also a precursor to and corresponds with hip pain. And again, it's because the psoas muscle is too tight.

According to *The Bone & Joint Journal*, persistent groin pain is becoming more common, even after seemingly successful total hip replacement surgeries (THRs). Recent studies have documented that up to 18 percent of THR recipients require femur resurfacing. One of the causes for this is iliopsoas tendinitis and impingement—which translates to a tight psoas! Just as we saw in the case of sciatica, if you have back issues that aren't dealt with, it can lead to the degeneration of cartilage on the inside of the hip socket and the need for hip replacement surgery.

The moral of the story? Many THR surgeries are successful these days, but if you have hip surgery and don't fix your psoas, you'll likely develop back problems later.

See DIY Remedies (starting with top three remedies, pages 130–35): Top three, lunge stretch (144–45). Cup GB 27, GB 28, LV 13, LV 14, GB 24, SP 16, CV 15, KI 20, and KI 21 (134–35, 165, 173–74, 176). Dredge LV 3 and GB 43 (166, 174). Foam roller on glutes, hips, and upper back (150–51). Foam roller or gua sha on outside of leg on GB 31 and GB 32 (153, 176).

10. PLANTAR FASCIITIS AND ACHILLES' HEEL

These conditions are also a byproduct of a too-tight psoas muscle.

Plantar fasciitis and Achilles' heel pain can obviously be caused by your calf muscle being too tight or wearing the wrong type of shoes for too long without proper support. This is one of the most common causes of heel pain. The pain shows up because of inflammation in the tendons and tissues that run across the bottom of your foot connecting the heel bone to the toes.

In my clinical practice, besides working on the heel and the calf muscle, I start off by working with the psoas muscle. When the psoas muscle is too tight, it restricts communication from the waist down to the feet and toes via the nerves and acupuncture meridians. Even if a client does not have back pain or back problems, when working with the psoas muscle to fix heel and foot problems, you will find that the muscle group will be very tight (even if the client has not been aware of it).

See DIY Remedies (starting with top three remedies, pages 130–35): Top three, lunge stretch (144–45), gua sha down from the lateral knee toward the medial ankle and Achilles' heel (183, 187). If you're a practitioner, gua sha on the back of the calf on the bladder channel itself (182). Foam roller on glutes, hips, and upper back (150–51). Foam roller or gua sha on outside of leg on GB 31 and GB 32 (152–53, 176).

11. KNEE PAIN

This condition is frequently a byproduct of lower back issues. It is said that the knee is stuck between the hip and the foot with nowhere to go and nowhere to hide.

There are many types of knee pain, and, believe it or not, your stomach influences the strength of your knees. The Stomach and Spleen are responsible for transforming and transporting food and fluid in your body. If there's an impairment in digestion, the pure fluids become impure and as a result turn into phlegm. Phlegm isn't just something that we find in our lungs or sinuses. It can be found in other places of the body as well. Thus, according to CCM, gout, infections, and certain types of arthritis are rooted in dysfunction of the Stomach and Spleen.

How does this relate to your back, you might wonder? One of the Spleen's functions is to control the muscles, and one of the muscle groups it controls is the psoas. So if you're not eating the right foods and/or you tend to worry a lot or are overly anxious, it can cause the synovial fluid in the knee to turn into phlegm, which causes pain.

Many times, knee pain shows up as the result of an injury, such as a ruptured ligament or torn meniscus. If the psoas is too tight, it can create a predisposition for these types of injuries, meaning that a deficiency or weakness comes first and, as a result, the person moves the wrong way and—voila! Injury. Obstruction of the belt channel (a horizontal meridian that circles the waist) via a tight psoas will also create a blockage of the three yin acupuncture meridians on the inside of the legs and feet as well as the three outside yang meridians of the legs.

The psoas muscle is like a belt. If that belt is too tight, it will cut off the circulation to whatever is below the waist. All six of these acupuncture meridians on both legs pass either around, behind, or over the top of the knee; that's why the knee becomes weak if the psoas is tight. A tight psoas will not only inhibit energy flow but will hamper nerve communication to the knees, feet, and toes, causing a weakness, or deficiency, that produces pain.

See DIY Remedies (starting with top three remedies, pages 130–35): Top three, gua sha on outside GB 32 to GB 33 or inside of the knee LV 9 (152–53, 176, 183). If you're a practitioner, gua sha on GB 40 and KI 10 (behind the knee; 179). Also gua sha inside the Liver and Spleen channel away from the knee (187). Only gua sha over these areas when marks from the previous sessions are gone. Light to medium cupping on UB 40, KI 10, LV 9, GB 33, ST 33, ST 34, SP 4, and SP 6 (179, 182, 183, 187, and see image below). Foam roller on glutes, hips, and upper back (150–52). Foam roller outside of leg on GB 31 and GB 32.

Stomach Meridian

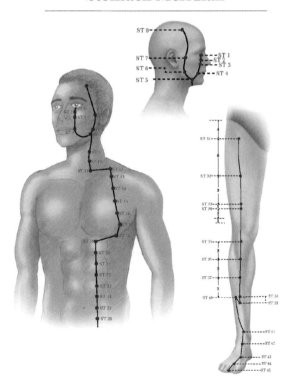

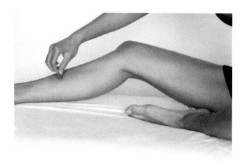

12. NUMBNESS OF FEET AND/OR TOES

Numbness, tingling, or pain in the feet and toes, including stabbing pain in one or more of the toes, is a common byproduct of any of the lower back, sacroiliac, and sciatica pain conditions listed above.

After the weightlifting injury mentioned earlier, once the cartilage in my hip had nearly healed, I started to develop pain in my big toe. This pain came and went. At its most severe, it felt like the bone was actually trying to break through the end of my toe! The lunge stretch, psoas stretch, and lying on tennis balls at specific acupuncture points fixed the problem.

When vertebrae compress the discs and impinge nerves exiting the spinal canal, it creates pain and/or numbness because some of these nerves reach all the way down to the toes.

Certain types of numbness, tingling, cold, or pain in the feet and toes can be a sign of other medical conditions as well. That's why it's really important to see your primary care physician if you're experiencing any of these symptoms in order to rule out other possible health issues.

On the milder end of the spectrum, numbness and tingling can be the result of shoes that are too tight or a bunion on your toe. More severe diseases that can cause numbness and tingling are diabetes, multiple sclerosis, Raynaud's disease, alcoholism, and peripheral artery disease.

See DIY Remedies (starting with top three remedies, pages 130–35): Top three, tennis ball press on UB 30, UB 34, UB 35, UB 53, UB 54, and GB 30 (146, 148–49). Tennis ball roll from upper back to middle back (147), lunge stretch (144–45), cupping GB 32, GB 33, LV 13, LV 14, ST 19, ST 20, KI 20, KI 21, CV 15, ST 33, ST 34, and LV 9 (173, 174, 176, 183, 186). Do not re-cup over these areas if there are still marks from the previous session. Light to medium cupping on UB 40 and KI 10 (179). Foam roller on glutes, hips, and upper back. Foam roller on outside of leg on GB 31 and GB 32 (150–51).

9

THE MIDDLE BACK, RIB PAIN, AND SIDE STITCH

You don't hear much about mid-back pain—that is, pain in the lower mid-section and thoracic spine area.

With pain in this region, usually you'll think something like "I have a rib out of whack" or "I have shortness of breath." You might feel pain whenever you pull something, lift your arm, or try to roll out of bed or when you lift something. At the time, you probably think you need to get an adjustment to help pop that rib back into place.

I thought the same thing one time and went to see my good friend the chiropractor. She popped that rib back in, and guess what? It popped out again—or at least I thought it did. What I realized over the years was that the rib *could* actually pop out, over and over. When that's the case, an adjustment is fantastic for resetting it, but if it keeps getting out of alignment, we have to look at what's going on inside the body.

This is because the true cause of what appears to be rib pain or a rib being out of place is actually an internal organ imbalance. Can you guess which internal organ it is? That pesky Liver.

In truth, it's not really pesky. It just gets to a point where it says, "You know, I'd love to process these toxins, I'd love to clear out the system, but I'm overwhelmed!" This happens because our livers are processing environmental and food toxins, then we pile emotional toxins like anger, frustration, rage, and resentment on top of that. At a certain point, the Liver Blood and Qi become congested.

MID-BACK 101

In this book, we are discussing issues with the lower lumbar, the thoracic spine, and the cervical spine. The thoracic spine tends to get overlooked. Most clients who come into my clinic will talk about lower lumbar issues but get confused between that and the mid-back area, or thoracic spine.

This chapter will help clear up that confusion.

So what and where is the thoracic spine? It starts below the collarbone and ends at the bottom of the rib cage. It is composed of 12 vertebrae, starting with T-1 at the base of the neck and ending at T-12 in the abdomen. It's the only part of the spine that's attached to the rib cage. It supports the neck and protects the spinal cord and soft tissues.

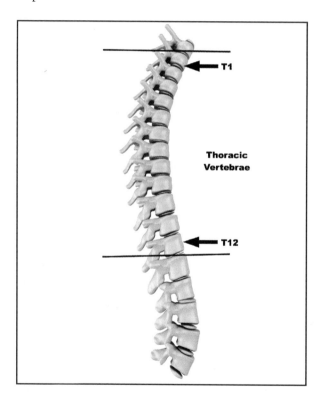

Thoracic spine pain, or rib pain, affects about 35 percent of the population every year. It can show up as diseases like osteoporosis (a condition in which the bones become porous and fragile), spinal degeneration, spinal stenosis, or osteomyelitis, an inflammation or infection of the bone.

The nerves of the thoracic spine control your arms, esophagus, heart, lungs, chest, larynx, trachea, gallbladder, liver, stomach, pancreas, spleen, diaphragm, kidneys, small intestine, appendix, adrenal system, colon, and small intestine. Therefore, mid-back conditions can be the root of or an extension of many diseases that affect these specific organs and their systems.

Anyone can experience mid-back and rib pain, but of all the Five Element typologies, Wood and Earth types are more prone to mid-back conditions.

Here's how you'll know.

DON'T IGNORE THESE WARNING SIGNS

There are warning signs that will let you know your Liver is out of balance before your back pain becomes severe or chronic. For example, you may have pain in the upper right or left quadrants of the rib cage, called the hypochondrium region. See image below. This refers to the upper third of the abdomen and rib cage and consists of the liver and gallbladder on the right side and the spleen and stomach on the left side.

If this pain persists, you should make an appointment with your primary care physician to rule out any chronic or deadly disease such as cancer of the liver, gallbladder, kidneys, stomach, spleen, pancreas, or intestines. Chances are, if you're not drinking too much and don't have gallstones, they won't find anything, but it's always better to play it safe.

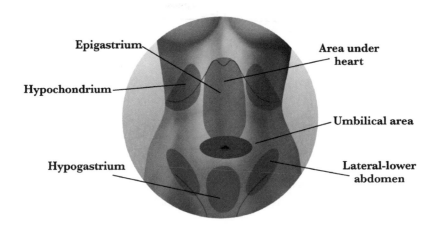

Another warning sign is if the area in the middle of your upper abdomen (at the base of the sternum) is painful or feels stuck, tight, bloated, or distended. This area is called the epigastric region. Once again, it's a good idea to have a complete blood panel done by your physician. This region houses the pancreas, and we want to be aware of possible pancreatitis and other similar diseases.

The liver stretches from the right hypochondrium region through the epigastric region and into the left hypochondrium region. It is a big organ and along with the intestines takes up a significant part of the abdominal cavity. Therefore, what we refer to as Liver Blood or Liver Qi stagnation can be the cause of discomfort in this entire area.

You may also have pain on your left or right side from the lower ribs up through the side of the rib cage. This is known as the lateral costal region. If you feel pain or distension in this area or if you experience nausea and vomiting, you'll want to really pay attention to it and talk to your physician.

As long as disease is ruled out by your primary care physician, we can look to Chinese medicine to help us determine why these areas are so uncomfortable. The cool thing about Chinese medicine is that we have many ways to assess or diagnose a situation.

One of our best forms of assessment is looking at the tongue. Did you know that our tongues tell us what's going on with specific internal organs in the present moment? It also tells us about past diseases and can provide insight into things like whether we're sleeping well. If there is stagnant blood in the Liver, the tongue may have a purple hue, especially along the sides.

We can also palpate the abdomen and feel for tender spots, particularly if they're over specific acupuncture points, such as Liver 13 and 14. These points give us immediate information about what is going on with the related organs.

The next thing we'll do is ask what other symptoms you have.

PHYSICAL SIGNS THAT YOUR LIVER IS OUT OF BALANCE

When the Liver gets out of balance and Qi or blood gets congested, you could have symptoms like the following:

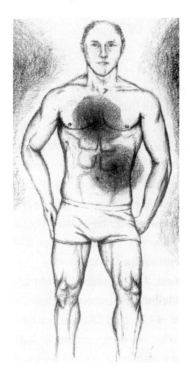

- Migraines

- Eye floaters

- Menstrual problems, cramping, PMS

- Moodiness, depression, explosive temper

- Neurological problems like facial neuralgia, Tourette's syndrome, eye tremors, or Bell's palsy

- Digestive issues like bloating, gas, colitis, constipation, diarrhea, Crohn's disease, or irritable bowel syndrome (IBS)

- Tendon and ligament issues, teeth grinding, and TMJ (temporomandibular joint) pain

These are a few of the symptoms that can be precursors of, or coincide with, the feeling that a rib is out in the middle back.

If you're experiencing these symptoms, one day you may wake up, reach for something high or bend over and suddenly realize, "Oh, I have a pain in the back of my rib here!" That's your Liver knocking on your back door and saying, "Listen to me, I'm at capacity, and we need to do some Qigong." You're probably under a lot of stress and/or feeling some resentment toward a person, situation, or institution. As a result, Liver Qi and blood have actually gotten stuck. This causes the Liver to expand and press on the ribs, which in turn causes pain and shortness of breath.

The Liver is most prone to disease in the spring. If you get springtime allergies, and/or if you have mid-back pain during this time of the year, that's your Liver raising a red flag. So what can you do to soothe the Liver?

QIGONG AND TAI CHI
FOR MID-BACK PAIN AND SIDE STITCH

The lymphatic system is an organ system located inside the spine. One of its main functions is to maintain fluid balance in the body. It also helps detoxify the blood and is one of the systems responsible for helping us fight off infection.

Qigong and Tai Chi are excellent practices to relieve rib pain and side stitch (exercise-related sharp abdominal pain) because the gentle movements and pumping actions aid the lymphatic system in moving fluids and detoxifying the blood. Nine times out of ten, rib pain or side stitch happens because Liver Blood and/or Liver Qi has been stagnant or because there's some type of Spleen dysfunction. Doing these movements will invigorate the lymphatic system and help cleanse the blood.

The best Qigong practices are the Liver cleansing movement, the Liver healing sound the Spleen cleansing movement, the Spleen healing sound, and massaging of the yang organs (see below). Additional Qigong exercises referenced in my first book, *Qigong for Self-Refinement* (soon to be republished as *Chris Shelton's Easy Guide to Emotional Well-Being with Qigong*, 3rd ed.), are also excellent practices that will support these main practices for rectifying rib and side stitch pain.

Do these exercises daily and make them a habit for the prevention of rib pain or side stitch:

1. THE LIVER CLEANSING EXERCISE

Bring the right palm face up to the right side of the body. Press the left palm forward as if you were trying to push something away from the body. As you pull the left arm and palm back, press the right arm and palm into the pushing-away position. At the same time, pull the left palm to the left side of the body, facing up. There should be a rolling effect of the palms as they pass one another midway through the movement. Your tongue should be pointing straight up on the roof of the mouth. You can do this practice each day, with between 9 and 36 repetitions at a minimum. If you want to get more from the practice, position your body to face east; this direction relates to the Liver and Gallbladder. The positive virtues of these organs, when in balance, are creativity, kindness, and acceptance. Balancing these organs will not only aid in preventing mid-back pain but will allow for greater emotional health as well.

2. THE LIVER HEALING SOUND

The great thing about healing sounds is that you can do them anywhere, from a seated, standing, or lying-down position. See chart on page 137.

Begin this meditation by imagining the breath filling up into the Liver and Gallbladder on the right side of your body. Imagine a green cloud rising up into the Liver and Gallbladder as you breathe in. At the same time, focus on something from the past or present that has created anger, frustration, resentment, or irritation. Feel it. Visualize who and what was involved. Then, as you exhale, make the *shuu* sound. Imagine the anger or resentment leaving like a dark cloud, going several feet away from the body and deep into the ground. Do this over and over, out loud if possible. Again, as you inhale, feel the forest-green cloud fill up into the right side of the body, and as you exhale, imagine your anger leaving like a dark cloud. If you're in public, it's okay to do the *shuu* sound under your breath. You can do this practice audibly or under your breath for 5 to 10 minutes at a time, whenever these emotions come up. Focus on different events or situations that make you angry.

3. THE SPLEEN CLEANSING EXERCISE

Stand in Wuji posture with your feet shoulder-width apart, shoulders relaxed and broad, tailbone tucked, pressing the crown point up. Place the tip of the tongue pointing downward behind the teeth. Imagine you're holding a beach ball between your abdomen and your right arm as you shift your weight onto the left leg. Begin to shift toward the right, inhaling as your body is centered and then exhaling as you imagine the beach ball transferring to the left arm (held between the abdomen and the left forearm) as you shift to the right. Exhale. Inhale again in the center and then, as you exhale, transfer this imaginary beach ball so that it rests between the right forearm and left torso. As you inhale, imagine a yellow or orange cloud filling up into the left side of your body where the Spleen is located. As you exhale, allow worry and anxiety to leave through the bottom of your feet and sink deep into the ground. Do this practice 9 to 36 times, allowing the positive virtues of peace of mind and centeredness to come into place.

4. THE SPLEEN HEALING SOUND

Begin this practice from a seated, standing, or lying-down position. Breathe into the left side of the body underneath the rib cage and imagine a yellow or orange cloud filling up this area. Focus on emotions of worry, pensiveness, and anxiety. Feel these emotions. Think about their cause in the past or present and who was involved. As you exhale, make the *huuu* sound audibly, allowing for the worry and anxiety to leave like a dark cloud, going several feet away from the body and deep into the ground. Each time you inhale, the yellowish orange cloud fills up deeper into the Spleen and Stomach. As you exhale, allow worry and anxiety to leave. You can do this practice audibly or under your breath for 5 to 10 minutes at a time, whenever these emotions come up. Allow the positive virtues of peace of mind and centeredness to take the place of worry.

5. MASSAGING THE YANG ORGANS

Begin this practice by standing in Wuji posture—feet shoulder-width apart, tailbone tucked, and chin tucked so as to raise the crown point on the top of the head. Relax your body. Bending your arms at the elbows, bring your forearms upward until your hands are shoulder height. Inhale through the nose into the lower abdomen. Keep the abdomen relaxed and allow it to expand as it fills up with air. Exhale and contract your abdomen, releasing the air as your arms swing down and then back up, using about 70 percent power (that is, let inertia help carry the arms on the downswing). As you inhale, bring your arms back up to shoulder height, and as you exhale, allow them to swing back down again. To make this into more of a mindfulness practice, you can imagine golden light filling up into your abdominal cavity as you inhale. Then as you exhale, imagine any toxicity from the Liver, Gallbladder, Stomach, Spleen, pancreas, or intestines releasing through the bottom of your feet and deep into the ground.

REMEDIES FOR MID-BACK PAIN AND SIDE STITCH

In addition to the exercises above, here are some of the best at-home healing techniques for mid-back pain.

1. CUPPING

When applying cupping techniques for side stitch and mid-back pain, it's important not to cup over the soft organs of the belly. If blisters come up under a cup or two on certain acupuncture points, do not cup over those areas again until they have completely healed. Do not re-cup over areas where there are still dark marks from past cupping. Sometimes, due to stagnation in the body, you may see a hint of where a cup was once placed. It's okay to cup over that area again.

> **Session 1:** Cup on LV 13, LV 14, and CV 15. Apply three to four pumps to the cup and leave on for 10 to 15 minutes (see pages 164–65, 174, and image directly below).

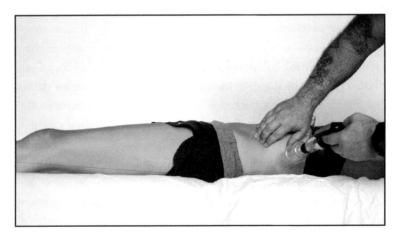

Session 2: Two to three days later, cup on ST 19, KI 22, GB 24, GB 25, and SP 16. Apply three to four pumps to the cup and leave on for 10 to 15 minutes.

Session 3: Once these areas have cleared up, you can mix and match cupping your acupuncture points. For example, you can do LV 13 and LV 14 in combination with ST 19 and GB 25.

2. GUA SHA

Another very useful technique is to gua sha some of the specific acupuncture points mentioned above. The main acupuncture points I use in the clinic are LV 13, LV 14, CV 15, GB 24, SP 16, ST 19, KI 21, and KI 22. Sometimes I gua sha the epigastric and hypochondrium regions right underneath the rib cage.

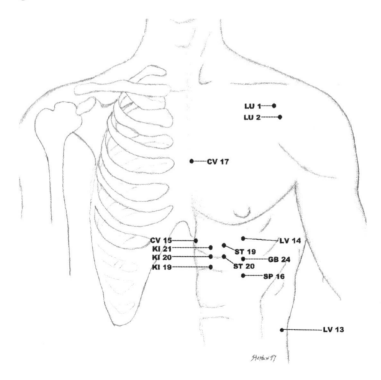

When doing gua sha on CV 15, I start from the base of the sternum and gua sha about one inch downward toward the belly button.

When doing gua sha on the other acupuncture points mentioned above, I normally start over the points and rub outward toward the lateral side of the rib cage, approximately half an inch.

Another powerful technique is to gua sha some of the specific points and then cup over the top. If you notice one or two drops of blood come up when you're finished, don't worry. This is normal, due to the amount of stagnation in the body.

3. ABDOMINAL MASSAGE

Abdominal massage is a very beneficial way to help to move blood, Qi, and fluids. Begin by applying coconut oil to the abdomen. Start at the belly button with one palm over the other. Rub in a circular motion outward, doing 36 rotations in total. During each rotation, move your hands farther away from the belly button and toward the lateral side of the rib cage and the base of the sternum. Note: Many times, constipation and diarrhea are caused by Liver and Spleen imbalances, so while you're alleviating your side stitch, you can also work to rectify these other two imbalances. If you suffer from constipation, you can use your mind's intent and circulate your hands in a clockwise rotation until reaching the lateral side of the rib cage and the base of the sternum. If you suffer from diarrhea, do the same practice but in a counterclockwise rotation.

Remember, any practice that helps bring balance to the Liver and Spleen will help heal and prevent back pain, especially mid-back, rib, and side stitch pain.

4. ACUPRESSURE

Apply acupressure to LV 3 in the web between the big toe and second toe. You can massage this point or apply coconut oil and rub down toward the inner base of the toenail on the big toe. Apply the same technique by massaging GB 43 between the pinky toe and fourth toe, about an inch from the web of the toes. See foot image on the next page.

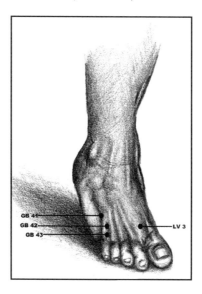

FOOD REMEDIES FOR MID-BACK PAIN AND SIDE STITCH

The following foods and drinks will help ease your mid-back pain.

1. HOT WATER AND LEMON ON AN EMPTY STOMACH

One of the best things you can do every single day is to start off with a four-ounce glass of hot water mixed with the juice of a whole lemon or lime and half a teaspoon of coconut oil. This will kick-start your digestion for the day and benefit your Liver and Gallbladder.

2. SHIITAKE STOCK RECIPE

To 8 cups of spring water, add:

2 cups shiitake mushrooms, sliced, with stems removed

2 celery stalks, minced

1 medium onion or a large leek

⅓ cup parsley, finely chopped

4 to 6 cloves of garlic, minced

3 bay leaves

1 tablespoon of ghee

$\frac{1}{2}$ tablespoon of sage

Sea salt or tamari to taste

Sauté the onion or leek and garlic in ghee. Combine all the other ingredients and bring to a boil. Cover and simmer for 45 minutes. Strain the stock. Save the mushrooms for other dishes and discard the other vegetables. Continue simmering the stock for an additional 15 minutes to reduce further and intensify the flavor.

3. CHRYSANTHEMUM TEA

Order chrysanthemum flowers online (Amazon, etc.) or go to your local herbalist. Add the dried flowers to a tea ball and steep for 10–15 minutes. Add some rock sugar (or *nabat*, as it is called in Persian culture) to the chrysanthemum flowers. It not only tastes great but can generally help clear Liver stagnation. Rock sugar, or *nabat*, has a different energetic property than regular sugar and is recommended in Chinese herbology for specific conditions. Chrysanthemum flowers also taste fantastic on their own. They have a gentle, cleansing effect on the body. Burdock root is beneficial as well.

4. SHIITAKE AND REISHI MUSHROOMS

If you have a hard time finding these mushrooms fresh, you can usually find them dried, especially online. You can also purchase them as an herbal supplement, pill, or tincture.

5. OTHER FOODS THAT BENEFIT THE LIVER

Tangerines, grapefruit, mint, fennel, ginger, small amounts of pickled vegetables, miso, soy sauce, mustard greens, asparagus, cabbage, artichokes, cauliflower, turnips, garlic, onions, kimchi, and vinegar

6. FOODS THAT BENEFIT THE SPLEEN

If you look at your tongue and see that it is large and flabby, with tooth marks on it, chances are you have a Spleen Qi deficiency or weakness. These are some of the foods and cooking methods that will help: Eat mostly organic vegetables, slightly sautéed or blanched. Avoid all cold and raw foods including salads, smoothies, and ice-cold drinks. Add more sweet potato, pumpkin, acorn squash, and spaghetti squash to your diet. Eat small amounts of organic grass-fed beef, chicken, turkey, and fish. Grains like basmati rice, quinoa, and oats are also good for you.

Foods to avoid: Excessive amounts of citrus, molasses, dairy, peanut butter, sugar, and chocolate.

DAILY HABITS FOR MID-BACK PAIN AND SIDE STITCH PREVENTION

Once you get your mid-back pain under control, make these lifestyle changes to help ensure that it doesn't come back again.

1. AVOID GREASY, FATTY, AND FRIED FOODS

The Gallbladder does not like greasy, fatty, fried foods or lots of fat in general, so cut out the unhealthy fats (animal fats) from your diet. You can add in more healthy fats like avocado, ghee, and coconut oil instead. Those are fantastic. Excess sugar and too many spicy foods can also disrupt the function of the Liver and the Gallbladder. Too many bad fats irritate them, causing the Liver to expand and create mid-back pain, or what feels like a rib out of place.

2. BE MINDFUL OF YOUR EMOTIONS

Emotions to pay attention to include stress, chronic stress, irritation, frustration, resentment, old anger, and not expressing your truth or not standing up and speaking your truth. People often want to project their paradigm or worldview onto others. If this happens to you, my recommendation is to speak up, stand up for your truth, and hold on to what you feel is correct and in alignment for you. This will help decongest the Liver.

3. USE THESE FENG SHUI REMEDIES

If you know your Liver needs some TLC, place the head of your bed on an east wall, if possible. You can also add green colors or live plants to your living and work areas. Artificial plants work but not as well as live ones.

Even pictures of trees and plants can be helpful. Rectangular shapes benefit the Liver, so adding square or rectangular sculptures to your environment will make subtle changes. If you know that your Spleen is deficient, add more yellow and orange tones to your environment. Paintings or pictures of deserts, fields, etc., are very beneficial. Yellow, orange, and square-shaped sculptures are also helpful for the Spleen—even something as simple as a square yellow candle.

10

NECK AND
SHOULDER ISSUES

Have you ever heard someone say, "That person is a pain in the neck!"? Well, it's actually true in certain situations, because most neck and shoulder pain is due to emotional events that affect the Heart. For example, if you have an argument or disagreement with a coworker, neighbor, family member, or spouse, a day or two later you may wake up with a stiff neck or a frozen shoulder.

Over 80 percent of adults over the age of 40 develop conditions like cervical spondylosis or cervical arthritis, and it is estimated that roughly 2 percent of the population suffers from frozen shoulder.

Conventional medicine uses steroidal injections, medication, and, finally, surgery to remedy the situation. But, just as in low and mid-back pain, neck and shoulder issues always come down to emotional stress in our lives. Chronic stress overactivates our nervous system, which causes a perpetual state of fight-or-flight accompanied by varying states of neck and back pain.

If conventional medicine specialists were to pause and ask their patients more profound questions about their emotional well-being and tension in their lives, they would probably help many more people before resorting to injections, anti-inflammatories, pain relievers, and surgery—which often don't even solve the problem in the long run.

On the other hand, it is true many people don't want to acknowledge that their emotional states can show up as disease or chronic pain. Much of this resistance has to do with cultural and family backgrounds.

This is where the foundations of Chinese medicine come in handy. Even if the client is unaware of potential emotional issues, we can help. This is because we have so many ways to diagnose or assess a situation. We can take the pulse, which tells us (short term and long term) what's going on inside the body. We can read the tongue, which tells us what's happening right here, right now and provides insight into past diseases. My favorite form of assessment is Chinese face reading. It's amazing, because every line and feature on a person's face tells the story of their personality, how they think, potential diseases at bay, and past traumas.

So let's dive into neck and shoulder pain.

CERVICAL SPINE 101

The area from the base of the skull down to the upper back is called the cervical spine. It's made up of eight vertebrae, starting with C1 at the base of the skull (also called the atlas bone because it holds the head up). The cervical spine area controls neck and head movement. It supports your head, which on average weighs about 8 to 12 pounds, and determines the relative position of the brain and spinal cord. Your cervical spine also influences the nerves that flow out of the vertebrae through the spinal canal and radiate down to the hands and fingers.

Each of the nerves that come out of individual sections of the cervical spine has a multitude of functions, including influencing the intracranial blood vessels, the eyes, the lacrimal gland (an almond-shaped gland behind each eye responsible for producing tears and lubricating the eye), and the parotid gland (located on each side of the mouth and ears, responsible for secreting saliva to the mouth, starting the digestive function, and controlling swallowing). These nerves also control the neck muscles, shoulders, elbows, arms, wrists, hands, and fingers. In addition, the cervical spine influences the diaphragm, the esophagus, the heart, the lungs, and the chest.

COMMON CONDITIONS OF THE CERVICAL SPINE

Here are some of the more frequent diagnoses for neck and shoulder issues.

1. CERVICAL STENOSIS

Cervical stenosis is caused by a narrowing of the spaces within the spine. This can put pressure on the nerves that travel through the spinal canal. When these openings constrict, they press on the nerves. As mentioned in previous chapters, you can have stenosis in other parts of the body as well, for example in the artery walls. If you have this condition, you may experience symptoms such as frequent head colds, fatigue, vision problems, sinus problems, migraine headaches, dizziness, allergies, sore throat, heart conditions, and high blood pressure.

2. CERVICAL ARTHRITIS

This is a basic term used to describe the degeneration of the discs and/or bones of the neck. As the discs dehydrate and shrink, signs of osteoarthritis develop, including bony projections along the edges of bones, called bone spurs. Cervical arthritis, or spondylosis, is very common and worsens with age. From my point of view, it's preventable if we properly deal with any emotional traumas that affect the heart as we age.

3. FROZEN NECK AND/OR FROZEN SHOULDER

These conditions are also known as *adhesive capsulitis*. They are characterized by stiffness and pain in the shoulder joint. Signs and symptoms typically begin gradually and worsen over time, although they can resolve on their own, usually within one to three years. The risk of developing frozen shoulder increases if you're recovering from a medical condition or procedure that prevents you from moving your arm, such as a stroke or a mastectomy. If you've had a mastectomy, chances are there are some major emotions surrounding it. So besides possible injury to the nerves during surgery, frozen shoulder may show up because of the related trauma.

Care for frozen shoulder in Western medicine consists of range-of-motion exercises and sometimes corticosteroids along with numbing medications injected directly into the joint capsule. In a small percentage of cases, arthroscopic surgery may be indicated to loosen the joint capsule so that it can move more freely. The problem with these treatments is that if the emotional issue isn't dealt with, the frozen shoulder will show up on the other side.

4. CERVICAL ATROPHY

Muscle atrophy is a wasting away of the muscles. In the case of cervical atrophy, this deterioration occurs in the neck and/or arm. Atrophy can happen when a disease or injury makes it difficult or impossible for you to move an arm. When the muscle starts deteriorating, it can be from lack of physical activity or the result of a channel pathology that creates deficiencies in the nerves and blood flow to the area. One sign of atrophied muscles is when one arm appears thinner but not shorter than the other arm. This will normally only happen when the blockage or impingement has been there for a while. The longer a blockage goes on, the more muscles will waste away.

We frequently see people with frozen shoulder; numbness or tingling of the arms, elbows, wrists, hands, and fingers; atrophy of the arm; cervical arthritis; or limited range of motion in the head and neck. All these issues result from the cervical spine pinching the nerves, usually because there's some type of stenosis, bulging, or herniated disc in the cervical spine.

COMMON CAUSES OF NECK AND SHOULDER PAIN

When a client comes in with neck and shoulder issues, I normally recommend that they see their primary care physician first for an MRI and/or an X-ray to rule out cancer of the spinal cord or the cervical spine itself. As long as it's not cancer (it's usually not), every single case that I see in my clinical practice comes down to the same thing—emotional trauma affecting the Heart and Lungs.

If you are doing jujitsu and someone knocks your shoulder out, or if you are pitching a softball or playing football and your shoulder pops out, that's obviously a physical condition. It would be the same with something like a car accident in which your shoulder was immediately dislocated and you couldn't move your head due to whiplash, for example.

On the other hand, if you walked away from that car accident feeling fine but a week or two later you experienced frozen shoulder or pain in the neck that radiated down into the arm and fingers, this would be directly due to your emotional response to the car accident. Some people might argue that the delay in pain showing up is the nervous system calming down or inflammation setting in. But in my experience, that's not the case.

If you wake up one morning and realize, "Oh, shoot, I can't turn my head" or "I have a limited range of motion in my shoulders," think back to what was going on a day, a couple of days, or maybe even a week before. Try to remember what was going on in your life that caused some type of emotional stress. That is actually at the root of the pain and discomfort.

In Chinese medicine, we view the acupuncture meridians like rivers. These rivers feed into lakes, which are our internal organs. Those lakes then feed into the three seas of energy referred to as the three Tan Tien. The lower Tan Tien is connected to our physical being, the middle Tan Tien influences our mental and emotional being, and the upper Tan Tien influences our spiritual connectedness. If you practice yoga or Ayurvedic medicine, the three Tan Tiens are comparable to the chakra system, which are seven energy centers along the center midline of the body.

If you consider the acupuncture meridians that stem from the hands, the upper chest, the shoulders, and up into the neck and face, all of them directly or indirectly connect back to the Heart and Lungs. Therefore, your pain could be caused by something like bottled-up resentment after a fight with your spouse, suppressed rage at your boss, lingering irritation at somebody cutting you off in traffic, or stress about financial issues. It could be that your dog died. Perhaps you had a sudden breakup or a loss in your life and the next thing you knew, you had a stiff neck.

Trust me, neck and shoulder pain always comes back to emotions that affect the Heart. The first step is to take inventory and really look at what is going on in your life.

A celebrity client came in with cervical arthritis. He had been suffering with it for three years, and you could see the arthritis on his X-ray. Our friends in Chicago had referred him to us, saying, "Look, before you have that surgery, why don't you fly out to San Jose and see our guy, Chris Shelton? He can help you." He did so reluctantly.

I started our session with some questions, one of which was, "What was going on in your life three years ago right before this showed up?" It's common for people to blame it on things like their mattress, their trainer recommending the wrong weightlifting routine, or their big dog who pulled on the leash too hard. This gentleman said that he thought it was stress from being on tour or the way he held his guitar on stage.

Then he paused and said, "You know what, Chris, two weeks before the cervical issues showed up, my horse died. My horse died, and I went back on tour. I did what everybody else does because we have to live our lives. I took care of business and moved on."

It's funny—he said that I got rid of his arthritis in 30 minutes. In reality, I just facilitated his body to release that trauma. Our session allowed him to make a mind-body connection. Acknowledging that this was a very painful time in his life helped with the healing process. You can see his interview with me on the @chrissheltonqigong YouTube channel.

Because my client didn't deal with the emotional components of losing his horse, what started out as neck and shoulder pain ended up as channel pathology, which occurs when there is a dysfunction of the acupuncture meridian itself. Over time, that channel pathology created a deficiency of nerve blood and fluid flowing through the affected area. It went on for so long that it started showing up as physical arthritis in his neck. When we suffer a great loss, such as an animal being put down or a loved one passing away, we still have to carry on with our lives. That is exactly what he did—and what most of us do. He took care of business and went back on tour, like nothing had happened.

I tell my clients that my job is not to force them into admitting they have emotional stressors in their lives. I simply present them with the opportunity to allow a deeper understanding of this mind-body connection.

Almost all the diseases I see (except for those that obviously result from a poor diet, drinking too much, not exercising, etc.) come back to the emotions. In Chinese medicine, your organs have a greater functionality than they do according to Western science. So when we look at the disease process for frozen shoulder or cervical issues, we look at the physiology but we also look at what's going on in the Heart.

What are you afraid to look at in your life now that you suddenly can't turn your head? Pause for a second and think about it. What are you afraid to acknowledge?

That's step number one—acknowledge it. Write it down; journal about it. These are great ways to energetically release trauma from the body.

If you took the Five Element Questionnaire and your primary element typology or weakest typology is Fire or Metal, you may be more prone to neck pain, shoulder pain, cervical issues, and numbness or tingling down the arm into the forearm, wrist, hands, and fingers. However, all of the element typologies can end up with cervical or shoulder issues because when your

Heart is affected emotionally by trauma, no matter how small or minor, it will cause the channels in the arms to become obstructed.

NECK AND SHOULDER PAIN AND YOUR FIVE ELEMENT TYPOLOGY

The main organs and associated channels that become obstructed and create deficiency or pain are as follows:

1. THE HEART

The Heart is the emperor or empress of the body. It dictates how much emotion is expressed or suppressed. If you cut off an emotion or don't express it appropriately, your body is going to alert you by creating inflammation in some form or another.

2. THE SMALL INTESTINE

The Heart works with the small intestine. When there are emotions affecting the Heart, they will often obstruct the Small Intestine meridian, which is the yang organ counterpart to the Heart. This acupuncture meridian flows from the outside edge of the pinky fingernail up the outside of the arm, through the shoulder girdle, up the neck, and into the face. When we see clients in the clinic, we resolve cervical issues or frozen shoulders by clearing and dredging the small intestine meridian, one of the main meridians in the neck.

3. THE PERICARDIUM AND THE TRIPLE BURNER

Another aspect of the Fire element is the Pericardium and what's known as the Triple Burner (or Triple Warmer). These acupuncture meridians also run from the fingers up through the shoulder and neck and into the face.

In fact, when we work with the Large Intestine meridian in the neck to fix these issues, people will often say they feel a burning sensation behind the ear. That's because the point we're working on stimulates the Triple Burner meridian flowing directly behind the ear and into the face.

So what's the Triple Burner? It's not an actual physiological organ. In fact, some clinical texts of Chinese medicine question whether the Triple Burner even exists. I tend to rely on the old classics, like the Yellow Emperor's *The Classic of Medicine*. This book states that the Triple Burner is not an actual physical organ but instead is an "energy net" within the visceral cavity that allows for all the internal organs to communicate properly with one another. The Upper Burner is referred to as the mist where the essence of our food, energy from our Kidneys, and the air we breathe produce the blood and Qi of our body. The Middle Burner is considered a maceration chamber where we digest our food and drink. The Lower Burner is thought of as the drainage ditch where waste is flushed out and the unused "good stuff" is sent back up to the chest where fluids enter in between the skin and muscles, etc.

The Pericardium is the sac that envelops and protects the Heart. One of its main functions is to protect the Heart from the pernicious influences of heat and fire as well as heat pathogens that can enter the body. It also takes the first hit from emotions that attack the Heart.

4. THE LUNGS

The Lungs are affected by the emotions of grief, sadness, sorrow, and disappointment. Guilt and shame fall in here as well. The Heart-Lung network is so closely intertwined that whenever you feel grief, shame, or guilt, it's going to attack the Lungs. Because the Lungs are so closely interconnected with the Heart, it is also affected.

The Lung acupuncture meridian starts in the lungs and larynx, emerges in the chest crease, flows all the way down the inner aspect of the arm to the thumb, and connects to the Large Intestine meridian. When the Lungs are affected by grief, sadness, or loss, this will obstruct the acupuncture channel for the Large Intestine meridian, which is bilateral for all the internal organs. This is what creates channel pathology, which in turn establishes deficiency and produces pain.

Once we calm down the nervous system, we can ease the mind and settle the spirit. Only then can we unwind, relieve stress, relax, and remove emotional blockages.

DIY QIGONG FOR CERVICAL, NECK, AND SHOULDER PAIN

Here are the top Qigong practices for healing neck and shoulder pain.

1. BRUSHING THE MERIDIANS

In this practice we use our hands to trace the meridians. This should harmonize and stimulate the flow of Qi. We move upward along the yin meridians (the inside of the body and limbs) as we inhale and we move our hands downward along the yang meridians (the outside of the body and limbs) while exhaling. Use a flat hand, palm facing the body. You may actually touch the body or you may keep your hand just above the body's surface. Clothes don't matter. Move at a speed consistent with your breath.

Preliminary

Start with the Three Regulations: steady breath, relaxed mind, Wuji posture (feet shoulder-width apart, shoulders relaxed, tailbone tucked, crown point rising).

Pull Down the Heavens (see below) three times. You may lightly bounce to relax and loosen the body.

Upper body

Begin with arms out to the side in a *T* position.

As you inhale, bring your hands together in front of your body and draw each hand up the opposite arm. That is, the right hand moves up the outside of the left arm while the left hand moves up the outside of the right arm.

At the shoulder, continue moving your hands up the sides of your head (arms will be crossed).

At the top of the head, uncross your hands.

Exhale as you let your hands flow naturally down the front of your body and then down the outsides of your legs.

Roll up on the balls of your feet as you flick your hands outward and say "*shuu*," releasing your breath with a sharp exhalation and dropping your heels down. Imagine that you are throwing any bad energy you have collected on your hands into the earth.

Next, lean over and put your hands on your feet, left hand on the left foot and right hand on the right foot. As you inhale, move your hands up the insides of your legs toward the groin.

After reaching the groin, cross your hands at the waist and move them up each side of your body into the armpits.

Exhale. As you do so, draw each hand down the opposite arm and down the inside of the forearms, then pull your hands apart, palms facing each other.

Repeat from step 1.

To end the practice, Pull Down the Heavens three times.

Pulling Down the Heavens

Start with feet hip-width apart, toes pointed forward, arms relaxed by your side. As you inhale, turn your palms up as you reach out and up toward the sky with both arms. As you exhale, face the palms toward the body as you bring the hands down the center midline. While you do this, imagine white light flowing through your body and deep into the ground.

2. THE HEART HEALING SOUND

Also referred to as the "dry cry" (see chart on page 137), this is by far the most important thing you can do to help clear out any cervical issues, neck pain, frozen shoulder, or tingling, burning, or numbness in the arms, hands, and fingers. You can do this practice anywhere—standing, seated, or lying down. Start by imagining that you are inhaling a pink cloud into your Heart. At the same time, remember any situations in your life that created pain or loss. If you can't come up with a specific memory, think about something from the present that bothers you. As you inhale, imagine the pink cloud filling up the entire heart muscle. As you exhale, make the *haaa* sound. Imagine and feel that circumstance leaving the body like a dark cloud, going several feet away and deep into the ground.

While doing this practice, if you find that you get a "stuck" feeling in your throat, also referred to as the "plum seed effect" in Chinese medicine, lift your chin as you make the *haaa* sound, and imagine the circumstance leaving from the throat like a dark cloud, going several feet away from the body and down deep into the ground. Do this practice daily for a minimum of 5 to 10 minutes. If you're in public and feel emotions come up, instead of suppressing them (which will only create more pain), make the sound under your breath. The cool thing is that no one will know what you are doing, and instead of bottling up your emotions, you are releasing them right on the spot.

3. THE HEART CLEANSING EXERCISE

Start this practice in Wuji posture, have your feet shoulder-width apart, shoulders relaxed and broad, tailbone tucked, pressing the crown point up. Place your hands in front of your lower abdomen as though you're cradling a baby. Start by turning your upper torso to the left. As you turn, raise your left arm and rotate the forearm to press the palm outward, with fingers horizontal. At the same time, brush the right arm across the body so that it's reaching to the left and under the left arm and have both palms facing out.

In traditional martial arts, this would be a classic "block and strike" type of move. When you've reached a comfortable extension, allow the arms to come back, returning to the starting position of cradling the baby. This time, allow for the right arm to come up in front of the forehead, palm facing out, with the left arm pressing underneath the right. As you inhale, imagine a pink cloud filling up into the Heart. On your exhale, imagine the loss or suffering leaving through the pinkies of both hands like a dark cloud, going several feet away from the body and down deep into the ground. (The inner corner of the pinky fingernail is where the Heart acupuncture meridian ends and connects to the Small Intestine meridian.)

4. THE LUNG HEALING SOUND

You can do this practice from a seated, lying-down, or standing position. I usually recommend starting off by standing in Wuji posture. Focus on any situation in your life that's created sadness, grief, sorrow, disappointment, guilt, and/or shame. Reflect on who's involved and what happened. As you inhale, imagine a white cloud filling up the Lungs. On your exhale, while making the *ssss* sound, imagine the grief and loss leaving like a dark cloud, going several feet away from the body and down deep into the ground. Do this practice daily, dredging up any old trauma that has caused you pain. You can do this practice for 5 to 10 minutes anytime you feel these emotions come up. If you're in public, you can make the sound under your breath. Instead of suppressing the emotion or waiting until you get home to deal with it, practice the *ssss* sound until you sense that the sharp edge of the feeling has lessened. This practice is also beneficial anytime you notice a "stuck" feeling in your throat.

5. THE LUNG CLEANSING EXERCISE

Start by standing in Wuji posture. Allow the arms to float up in front of the body to shoulder height, palms facing down. While inhaling, imagine a white or silver cloud filling up into the chest. Spread your arms out to the sides with palms down, as though you're opening curtains (this movement expands the chest). Turn your palms in and, while exhaling, bring them back to the front center of your body, close to the chest. Imagine any grief, sadness, sorrow, or disappointment leaving like a dark cloud, going several feet away from the body and down deep into the ground. Do this practice daily, focusing on traumas that have led to grief and loss for you. Please note that it is normal for the same situation or circumstance to come up over and over. This is because emotions have to be released in layers.

6. THE WHITE PEARL MEDITATION

Start this practice in a standing, seated, or lying-down position. Place your hands, one on top of the other, over the lower abdomen about one inch below your belly button. As you inhale, imagine a mystical white pearl expanding and enveloping your entire lower abdomen. As you exhale, imagine a white light radiating around the waist to the Kidneys on the lower back opposite your belly button. Each time you inhale, the pearl gets brighter and brighter. As you exhale, feel the warmth and the white light radiate around the waist to the Kidneys. Do this practice daily for at least 5 to 10 minutes. (We have this meditation available for download on iTunes and Spotify. It's a great practice for grounding yourself after clearing and working through the various emotions.)

FOOD REMEDIES FOR NECK AND SHOULDER PAIN

Although there's no specific diet to help prevent or cure neck and shoulder pain, there are simple do's and don'ts that can expedite the healing process. The common things to avoid are greasy, fatty, or fried foods; sugar; excessive amounts of meat and dairy; and the overconsumption of alcohol, processed foods, and cold or raw foods. Whenever possible, avoid eating foods that are genetically modified, sprayed with pesticides, or injected with antibiotics.

The primary way to slow the aging process as well as cut back on inflammation of the cervical spine and shoulder, is to eat more steamed vegetables. Vegetables should make up about 40 to 60 percent of our daily diet, and steaming them is best because it aids our body's ability to absorb the nutrients. Steamed vegetables are easier to digest because the stomach does not have to heat them up to assimilate them. During the summer when it's warmer outside, it's okay to have more salads, especially kale or spinach. Other vegetables that will benefit your daily rotation are brussels sprouts, broccoli, and onions.

Cooking with herbs like turmeric, cayenne pepper, dill, mint, and ginger is great for fighting off inflammation. Carry around snack baggies of unsalted sunflower seeds, almonds, pumpkin seeds, and walnuts; add dried goji berries or blueberries. Some of the best anti-inflammatory fruits are raspberries, strawberries, peaches, blackberries, blueberries, cherries, apples, pears, nectarines, apricots, plums, and pomegranates. It's best to eat three to four servings per day (a serving is one medium-sized piece of fruit).

Take care to avoid eating too much red meat or chicken. Based on your constitution, animal protein should make up no more than about 10 percent of your diet. When we evaluate food in Chinese nutrition, we look at the energetic properties and what organ or organ systems they affect. Energetically, chicken is the hottest of all meats. That's because chickens produce a lot of eggs and it takes heat to make those eggs. So if you have inflammation, which of course is hot, overeating chicken could aggravate the situation. Also, pay attention to how the animal was raised and slaughtered. I usually recommend free-range chicken and grass-fed beef. And knowing that there was compassion and love for the animal when it gave its life for us is important. That's why I recommend eating kosher or halal meat whenever possible.

Saltwater fish is not only good for inflammation but it has a lot of healthy omega-3 fats, which are excellent for brain health. The smaller the saltwater fish, the better for you, because they normally don't contain as much mercury as larger fish, which are higher up on the food chain and have consumed many smaller fish and therefore accumulated more mercury. Some of the fish I recommend are sardines, salmon, cod, herring, and mackerel. I advise eating shellfish sparingly because most shellfish are energetically hot, which can aggravate inflammation.

Adding other healthy fats to your diet such as coconut oil, avocado, and ghee will also help you lower inflammation and promote a healthy internal environment that supports the healing process.

DAILY REMEDIES FOR NECK AND SHOULDER PAIN

Make these practices regular habits to prevent neck and shoulder pain from recurring.

Practicing Qigong daily: Start or end your day with 20 to 30 minutes of Qigong. You can follow follow my channel @chrissheltonqigong on Youtube. There I have a free 30-Day Qigong to Better Health course that follows along with my first book. Or better yet, join us for daily workouts in The Qi Club at www.theqiclub.com.

Lying on tennis balls: Lie with a single tennis ball on the SI 11 acupuncture point in the center of the scapula and on UB 43 (see image below and on page 147) at the bottom of the shoulder blade between the shoulder blade and spine. This is a meeting point of the Heart, Stomach, and Liver and influences the shoulder as well. Also, lie with a tennis ball under your hip on UB 54 (see image on page 149). Shoulder pain is often accompanied by hip issues on the opposite side of the body.

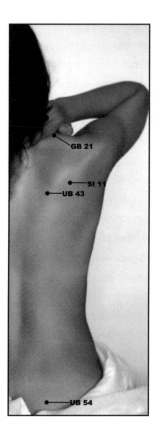

Massaging LI 4: Massage the web between your thumb and the pointer finger. This acupuncture point helps clear the Large Intestine meridian that flows through the neck and into the face. You can massage these points on both hands. After massaging for a minute or so, squeeze the point and imagine releasing the pain out of the neck or shoulder. Grab your pointer finger with the opposite hand and imagine the pain leaving through the tip of the finger. Do this practice daily for two to five minutes.

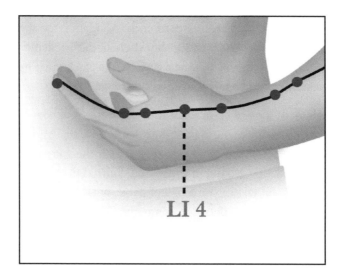

Massaging HT 9: With your thumb pressing on the inner lower corner of the pinky fingernail, where the Heart acupuncture meridian ends, close your eyes and imagine a pink cloud filling up your Heart. As you exhale, make the *haaa* sound and imagine any grief, sorrow, or negative feelings leaving out through the pinky nail. Do this practice daily for five to ten minutes.

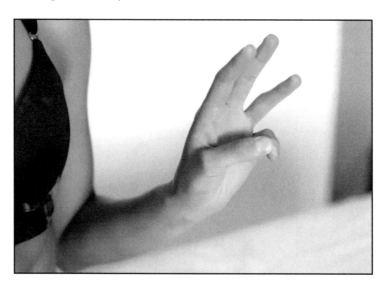

Neck rotation: From a seated or standing posture, slowly and gently rotate your head in a clockwise direction. As the head comes forward, imagine and feel the shoulders pulling forward and the back rounding. As your head rotates to the back, open up the shoulders and the chest, encompassing the whole upper back and shoulder girdle. After three to nine rotations in a clockwise direction, repeat in a counterclockwise direction.

Journaling: At the end of each day, take an inventory of how your day went. Write down any and all injustices or events that occurred that upset you. Be as detailed as possible. If there are past injustices circulating around in your mind, journal those out as well. I recommend writing on a pad of paper with a pen as opposed to typing it on your phone or computer. There's a greater energy exchange and release from your body to the pad of paper when you write.

ACUPRESSURE AND CUPPING TECHNIQUES FOR NECK AND SHOULDER PAIN

Here's how to use acupressure and cupping to relieve your neck and shoulder issues.

Cup LU 1 and LU 2 bilaterally on the upper chest in the shoulder crease (where the shoulder meets the chest) using three to four pumps. Leave on for no more than 10 or 15 minutes.

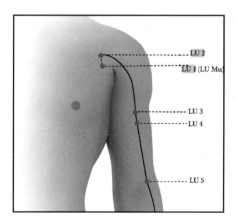

Cup GB 21 on the highest point of the trapezius muscle on the top of the shoulder. Use three to four pumps and leave on for no longer than 10 or 15 minutes. This point is contraindicated for pregnant women. See image below.

Cup SI 11 and SI 9 SI 11 is in the center of the shoulder blade. This is the connecting point for the Heart. There may or may not be a knot at this point, but it will be tender. The SI channel goes up the side of the neck to your cheek and ends in front of the ear. This is a tricky technique to do on yourself, so you might need someone else to help you reach it. Most cupping sets come with an extension hose, which allows you to reach these areas a little more easily. Apply three to four pumps to these points and leave on for no longer than 10 or 15 minutes.

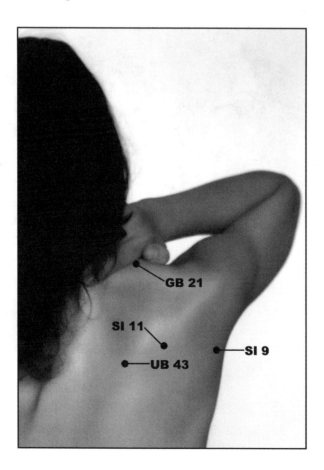

Gua sha CV 17 This is a very tender acupuncture point on the center of the sternum, which is a direct connection to the Heart and Pericardium. Apply coconut oil to this area and use a coin or a gua sha tool. Rub vigorously over the points in a downward direction toward the belly button. Please note that the gua sha area should be about half an inch to an inch long. See images below and on page 197.

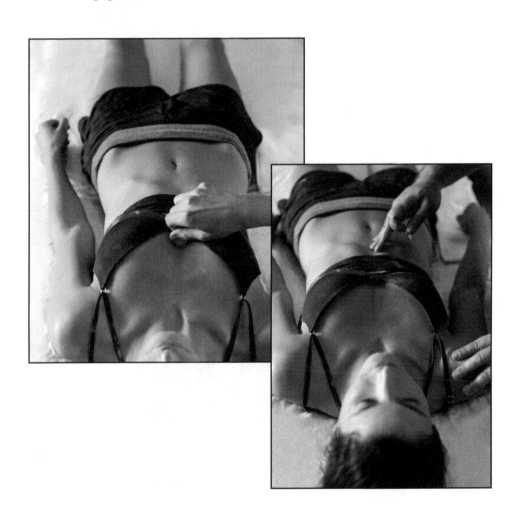

Gua sha LU 1 and LU 2 These acupuncture points are directly connected to the Lungs. Apply coconut oil and begin rubbing (using a coin or a gua sha tool) over both points, rubbing outward toward the side of the chest and into the armpit. The area being worked on should be no more than one or two inches wide. This might be a tender point, and the amount of trauma and grief that you've been holding on to can make it much more tender. It may be easier to have a practitioner do this technique. For a more profound release, you can add a cup to the LU 1 and LU 2 points as well.

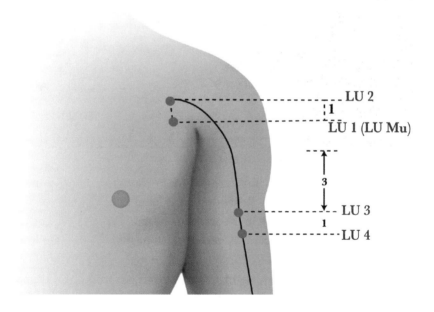

LU 2

1

LU 1 (LU Mu)

3

LU 3

1

LU 4

Gua sha LI 15 and GB 21 These acupuncture points have an indirect influence on the Heart and on the shoulder girdle (see image below and on page 153). Apply oil and, using a coin or a gua sha tool, begin rubbing from the base of the neck over these points and down toward the elbow.

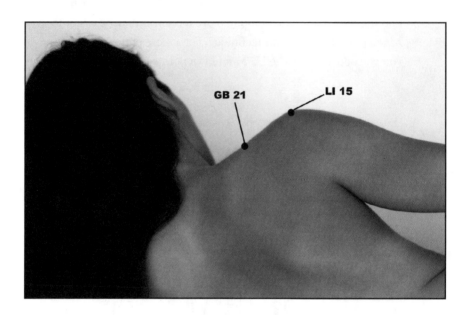

LI 18 and LI 17 press and release These two acupuncture points will likely be tender. Start by pressing into LI 18 on the side of the neck (LI 18 is closer to the jaw and above LI 17) on the opposite side of where the cervical issue or frozen shoulder is manifest. Nine times out of ten, chronic pain is rooted in the opposite side of the body. As you press firmly, rotate your head from left to right for one full rotation. Make the heart sound (*haaa*) as you exhale. As you inhale, imagine a pink cloud filling up the Heart. On your next exhale, imagine any grief or sorrow leaving like a dark cloud floating out several feet away from the body and down deep into the ground. After doing six to nine rotations with the head moving side to side, pressing on this point, move about half an inch down to LI 17 and do the same thing. Then move to the opposite side of the body and repeat on both of these points.

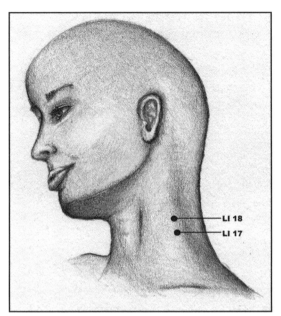

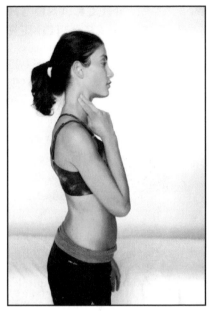

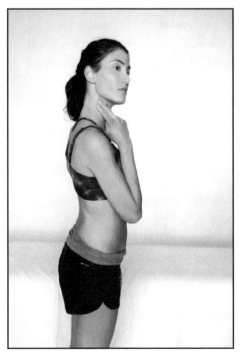

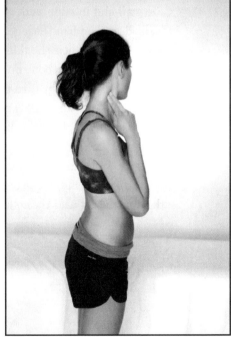

NECK AND SHOULDER: ACUPRESSURE FOR PRACTITIONERS AND SELF-ADMINISTRATION

LI 17 and LI 18 Press: If you are a practitioner, have the client sit on a chair or on the very edge of a massage table. Tuck one arm behind the lower back and have them rest it on the chair or table. This is the side on which you will be pressing on LI 18 and LI 17 first. As you press, have your client turn their head from left to right in one full rotation. Depending on the severity of the situation, this may be very painful and challenging for them to do. The more they can push themselves to try to rotate their head into your fingers, the more relief they will feel. They may even notice that when you start to press on LI 17, they get a shooting or burning pain down to the shoulder girdle and into the arm, possibly to the fingers.

Adjusting the Bicipital Tendon Technique: Have the client stand perpendicular to a wall, with their shoulder dropped and relaxed and leaning against the wall and the opposite shoulder turned in at about a 90-degree angle. Turn the head so their ear is against the wall and in alignment with the shoulder that's against the wall. Place their hand flat against the wall. Stand behind the client and reach over their shoulder. Press in and up with your fingers just under the collarbone on KI 21, until you find a tender spot. Have the client slowly turn their hand clockwise, keeping their shoulder against the wall. Then have them turn their hand back flat onto the wall. Find another tender point near the collarbone, and repeat the process.

If you feel that the tendon might be out, you can do this technique on yourself. Use the opposite hand to find tender points on the upper chest near the collarbone.

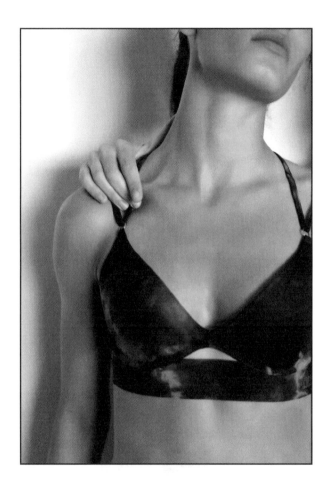

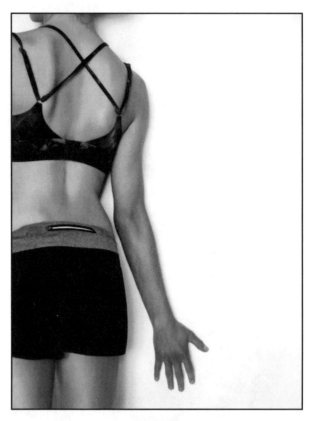

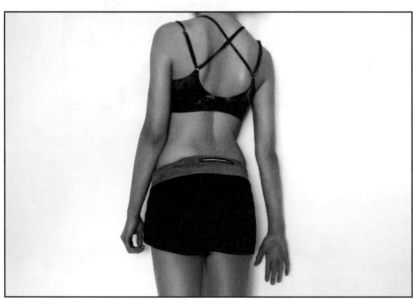

If you complete the LI 18 and LI 17 press and your client still has pain or limited range of motion, gua sha those specific acupuncture points. Ask the client where the pain has moved, because it will migrate from point to point and channel to channel. I sometimes joke that we have to chase the pain out of the body, but it's the truth.

With the client seated, press with thumbs or elbows on SI 9 and SI 11. Press these points until it hurts. Have them make the *haaa* sound, then brush down their arm. If you know the particular emotion that is involved, make the corresponding organ healing sound. Be especially gentle with the elderly, children, and immunocompromised people.

Gua sha the GB channel from GB 20 to GB 21. The GB channel runs up the back of the neck and terminates in the face (see page 219).

▪ 11 ▪

CONTINUING
YOUR HEALING JOURNEY

Congratulations on making it this far!

You are truly becoming your own superior doctor. You now have the tools to transform pain and suffering into vibrant health. As Lao Tzu said, "A journey of a thousand miles begins with a single step."

Wherever you are on your journey, whether you're an expert who has tried many different remedies to live a pain-free and balanced life or a novice who has just begun their search, picking up this book will help you on your journey.

The biggest takeaway I want you, my reader, to get is self-empowerment.

I want you to become so aware of your body through these ancient Qigong practices that you can ward off disease and pain before they set in. I want you to know that if you are suffering from any of the issues mentioned in this book, you can and will be able to transform that pain into wisdom and the ability to live the life you were designed to live.

In this book, I've introduced you to the philosophies of classical Chinese medicine with a modern approach. I've given you some very basic anatomy and physiology to help you understand how the body moves and functions. I've explained how integrating Eastern and Western approaches is essential in understanding how the body and mind function.

In the meantime, you've learned a lot:

- Your emotions, when not processed properly, get stuck in your internal organ systems and show up as chronic pain and disease.

- Your environment plays a major role in how you feel and in the discomfort and discord that shows up as a result of unfavorable environmental factors.

- Your relationships with family, friends, and work can affect you physically.

- When you are not in alignment with the seasons, it can manifest as disease, and those external climatic conditions can appear inside the body, showing up as fire, heat, dampness, dryness, and wind.

- Food has energetic properties and affects people differently. A food that is considered healthy can benefit most people and yet have certain properties that actually cause harm in other people.

- Certain colors, flavors, and directions can benefit our internal organs and, remarkably, help relieve pain.

- Some conventional, functional movement techniques and stretches will contribute to healing your pain.

- Cupping, gua sha, and moxibustion can create changes in the body when placed over specific acupuncture points and channels.

But the most valuable tools I am giving you are the simple, yet effective, gentle movement and meditation techniques found in the Qigong practices.

Take your time with this book. There's a lot to digest.

If you're currently suffering, go to the section of the book that teaches specific remedies that will help relieve your pain right away. Then I recommend going back and diving deeper into the etiology (or origins) and the foundation of what creates pain and disease in the first place.

I must emphasize that looking at your mental/emotional state, past traumas, and day-to-day experiences while using the Qigong practices (to help rid your body of those negative energies and experiences) is really important for obtaining vibrant health.

Also, recognize that the emotional pain and suffering we go through in our lives is there to help us awaken, learn, and expand. As we let go of negative experiences, we gain wisdom.

We can then share our stories and triumphs with others to help them on their journeys. I think it's important not to go to your grave holding on to what you've been through in your lifetime. It's especially important not to identify with your suffering, pain, and story. Use your story to uplift others.

In my 20+ years of clinical practice, I have helped thousands of people regain their health and transform pain into happiness. It's been such a blessing to be able to witness the transformation of so many, and I can tell you from the bottom of my heart that when you apply these simple techniques to your life, you can be pain free!

One client I worked with, Patty, came to me after dealing with severe back pain for more than 10 years. I could see the suffering on her face. Three years before coming to see me, she had had lower back surgery and was bedridden for almost a year. She was in more pain than before the surgery. In our session, we went through some of her history and I administered the techniques described in this book. I had her get up and walk to see how she was feeling, and as she was walking, she started to cry. I got nervous, thinking that I injured her. I asked her what was wrong. She said, "It's not what's wrong, it's what's right. This is the first time I have had no pain in over 10 years!"

My own journey led me to the practice of Qigong and Chinese medicine. The same practices I've taught you in this book cured me of my debilitating back injury over 30 years ago—and they've helped me keep my back healthy and strong ever since.

I was determined. I did not believe the physicians who said that I wouldn't be able to walk or compete in martial arts again. I proved them wrong—not only to fulfill my own destiny but to share this valuable information with you.

So what are your next steps?

- Sign up for our email list at www.sheltonqigong.com. We send out weekly tips and techniques to help you maintain health, vibrancy, and happiness.

- Consider joining our Qi Club (theqiclub.com) every Wednesday from 8:00 to 8:50 a.m. Pacific time, for live Qigong classes on

Zoom with other health-conscious people like yourself from around the world. On-demand videos are also available for those who cannot attend live.

- If you see the value and have felt the results of these practices, I strongly encourage you to consider signing up for our Level I Qigong Teacher Training Program at www.qigongteachertraining.com.

- Note that not everyone who takes the Qigong Teacher Training program wants to teach Qigong. If you do want to teach, we'll prepare you for that, but we've found that many students take this comprehensive Qigong training program simply to cultivate and understand themselves at a deeper level and to live their best lives.

- I also encourage you to subscribe to my YouTube channel, @chrissheltonqigong, and follow me on X, Facebook, and Instagram @chrissheltonqigong. You can also find me on TikTok @chris_shelton_qigong.

Thanks again for your love and support and for being the change that you want to see. I love being part of a community of like-minded individuals who are aware of the value of this one life. This book will help you learn how to preserve it.

May you be at peace and be happy. I'll Qi you later!

Chris Shelton

■ ■ ■

ACKNOWLEDGMENTS

There is not one successful person, past or present, who made it to where they are without the help and guidance, directly or indirectly, from a team of other people and from God. This book has been in the making for several years now—but to even to begin to write it, there was a series of events and people who influenced or created opportunities for me to get to this point. Therefore, I have to give the first acknowledgment to the all-knowing Oneness, also referred to as God or the Tao. I make this statement not as though I'm talking to a physical person but with the realization that, without God and accessing its greatness in my life and shining through as spirit, none of this ever would have come to fruition. God gave me the opportunity that all people have, and that is to find my life's purpose and, within that, harness the power of free will to co-manifest with God all the great accomplishments that come from serving thousands of people around the world. With God, I have the strength, the will, and the perseverance to overcome all obstacles and naysayers that didn't believe that I could make it.

The first person I'd like to thank is my wonderful wife, Parisa. She has been in the trenches with me since 2010. I say "trenches" because, after we first met, it seemed like many outside forces, including family, were obstacles in our path together. She has unselfishly fought the fight with me and has helped me blossom in many ways. Not only is she a nurturing stepmother (an *amazing* stepmother, that is) to my four kids, she's helped build the brand that I started in 2001, the Morning Crane Healing Arts Center. On top of that, within the last few years, we've started a few more brands: Shelton Qigong, Qigong Teacher Training, and, during the pandemic, The Qi Club. I always said that for a woman to be with me, she would have to be a strong individual, and that's who Parisa is. I love working with her, and appreciate that she does a lot of the back-end work for our business. She is the beacon of light that shines and gives me strength, especially when I'm on stage. She is loving and compassionate and really cares about our mission and community. But what I love the most about her is that what you see is what you get. There is nothing fake about this woman, and I'm grateful that we are on this journey together.

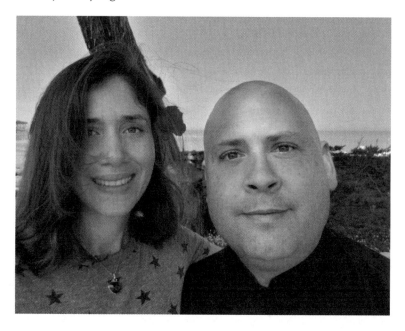

Next are my teachers. I am thankful to the person who introduced me to Qigong and Medical Qigong, Arnold Tayam. To my Sifu, Tony Wong, I am forever grateful. You took me in as a student and pushed me to become a Taiji practitioner. When I first met you at Rengstorff Park in Mountain View, California, I had been practicing what I thought was traditional Chen Tai Chi. I got about halfway through the form when you stopped me and said, "Chris, you obviously have some Tai Chi principles, but this is not traditional Chen Style Tai Chi. If you want to study with me, you have to start from the very beginning!" Discouraged, because I had just spent 11 years studying with another instructor, I followed your lead. As a result, I got to witness the true essence of traditional Chen Family Tai Chi Chuan. You gently guided and supported me while I was competing and giving public demonstrations with your team, and you are the catalyst of my growth and that of the Morning Crane Healing Arts Center. You've openly shared your heart, knowledge, and wisdom with me, and I'm grateful that you are my friend.

To my acupuncture teacher, Esther Su, I completely credit the success in my remedy strategies with clients to the private studies that I did with you for about two and a half years. You also saw my eagerness to learn and took me into your private practice. You taught me the ancient system of Tung style acupuncture. Even though I had finished a four-year Medical Qigong program with a lot of emphasis on the foundations of Chinese medicine, I humbly realized how much I did not know or understand. You had a way of teaching that made it easy for me to comprehend while implementing the deep philosophies from your teacher on Confucianism and Taoism. Though I didn't finish my studies with you, what I gained was immensely valuable. You taught me that the principle of Tung style is that you don't have to stick 100 needles in someone. Instead, you find the most powerful points and go after those. The development of strategies that I'm utilizing in this book and others are completely based upon your teachings. It's been a divine gift to become your friend and to tap into some of your deep wisdom.

Next is the Ni family. I started studying the Taoist teachings of Grandmaster Hua Ching Ni about 28 years ago. As a result, I got to look at what becoming egoless meant while cultivating the deeper meaning in the passages from your books, as well as how life force energy, or Qi, manifests in so many ways—from our spiritual cultivation to our health, our environment, and finally to our interconnectedness with all things. I had the privilege of being part of many workshops at Yo San University in Los Angeles and have had the privilege of taking classes with your sons, Dr. Mao and Dr. Tao. Words can't even describe how fortunate I've been to be able to listen to lectures from two of this country's greatest acupuncturists and physicians with the accumulated knowledge of 38 generations of Chinese and Taoist masters. One of the highlights of my career was being honored to do a Facebook Live workshop with Dr. Mao on the principles of Five Element philosophy. I especially appreciate his generosity in allowing me to share his family tradition in my teachings and writings. In fact, a lot of the philosophy of yin and yang and the Five Elements comes from Ni family traditions.

I am grateful to and sincerely thank Dr. Nancy Bergmann. Dr. Nancy helped to heal my back after my martial arts injury almost 30 years ago. If I hadn't met her, who knows if I'd be walking today. It's because of Dr. Nancy that I've been able to work and study with all the people I've listed above. She really is the foundation of my journey, and I employ her attitude toward healing in my practice every day. Some of the techniques used in this book are directly from Dr. Nancy Bergmann, and it was because of her that I was able to meet Liz Koch, the master of the psoas muscle. Dr. Nancy taught me foundational craniosacral techniques, dietary techniques, and functional movement techniques that I utilize in clinical practice today. Some of those techniques are listed in this book and upcoming books. What I love most about Dr. Nancy is her wisdom, her skill set, and her no-nonsense approach. I appreciate anyone that can tell you how it is and still care for you at the same time.

Shasta Tierra. After I finished my first four years of Medical Qigong, I came down with a flu bug that almost killed me. I was sick for almost a year! As a result, I ended up with other health problems. It was almost like the universe was saying to me, "Okay, Chris, if you think you know so much, fix yourself!" I had gone through everything in Western medicine, but nothing was working. Through working with Shasta, I was able to heal myself. During the process, she educated me as to what was going on and described her remedy strategies. Some of those healing techniques I use in my daily clinical practice and some will be taught in my upcoming books. Although it's been many years, I appreciate the friendship we had and her true spirit of just being herself.

Master Mark Johnson taught me the importance of feng shui according to your constitutional typology. I appreciate Mark's deep knowledge of and wisdom about classical Chinese medicine, Chinese astrology, Qigong, Tai Chi, and feng shui. I also appreciate Mark's straightforwardness and witty sense of humor. I've enjoyed the opportunity to be a judge with him at the UC Berkeley Chinese Martial Arts Competitions throughout the years.

There have been many other teachers that I've had the opportunity to work with who helped shape the person I am today. Some of my teachers are now my students and my clients. Through them, I've been able to grow and to learn, and I am grateful for every one of them.

Coach Cung Le has played an important role in helping promote my healing practice. Besides being my fight coach, friend, and client, Cung helped me secure some major publicity. Thanks to Cung, I've been on *Showtime, NBC Sports*, the UFC, and Vietnamese television from Los Angeles. As a result of the interview on Vietnamese television and the icon that Cung is in the Vietnamese community, I have a big following as "Cung's Doctor." This is what prompted us to publish my first book, *Qigong for Self-Refinement: Total Health with the 5 Elements*, in Vietnamese.

It was through Cung that I was introduced to my friend Eric the Trainer, the Hollywood physique expert. Eric had an enormous impact on helping me spread the art of Qigong and the healing practice I've developed. Eric pulled me into many of his public appearances. He was quite possibly one of my biggest megaphones. Because of Eric, I have been able to touch more lives while meeting some of the world's most talented and amazing people. He had an enormous heart and was a lighthouse for anyone he came in contact with. Because of him, I got to work with Maria Shriver and the Special Olympics, go on tour with Def Leppard, present at the Fit Expos, work with Quest Nutrition, and present at the International Chefs Conference. Unfortunately, Eric left us too soon, passing away on Thanksgiving morning in 2022. He was a true friend who unselfishly gave of himself, and I'm forever grateful to have had him in my life.

Tae Bo creator Billy Blanks has been a loyal supporter and friend who believes in me. Billy is a living illustration of what hard work, dedication, and compassion can do for the world. He's a man of authenticity and faith. Besides his friendship and support, I'm thankful that he introduced me to Christ and, as a result, our bond and friendship has grown deeper.

Vicki King is someone who had an indirect but powerful role in helping me launch my healing career. When I was a meat manager for Safeway, Vicki was a store manager and a big advocate for me. She helped me by working with supervisors and other store managers to allow me the opportunity to cut back my hours while I was building my clinical practice and the Morning Crane Healing Arts Center. Back in the day, by union contract and company policy, meat managers could not work less than 40 hours per week. Because of Vicki, I was able to go into shops that were struggling and help them pull up their profits while I got to dictate my own schedule. The last couple of years before I retired from the industry, I was working the minimum number of hours per week to keep my health benefits, only 20 hours. This was unheard of in the industry at the time. It goes to show you that when you're on the right path, God shows up and things just magically work out!

Next is my father, James Shelton. The Johnny Cash song "I Walk the Line" describes my personality. If it weren't for Qigong, who knows if I'd be alive today. Because of this extreme nature of mine, my father picked up the slack more than once and helped me out tremendously with my kids while I was working long days building my clinical practice. At first, he didn't really understand what it was I was striving for. After a few years, he ended up becoming a client of mine as well as a graduate of my Qigong Certification program. He also supported me by taking all the other classes I offered, from feng shui to Chinese face reading.

Ultimately this book would not have come to completion without the skillful eye of our line editor, Nichole Gates. She thoroughly went through the manuscript and made corrections and reformatted, and reorganized the information to make it easier for the reader. On top of being super talented, she's a beautiful spirit and has been easy to work with.

A true gift sent from the heavens is our entertainment and contractual lawyer, David Garfield Roland. He showed up in our life when my team tried to take over a 15-minute short documentary that my wife and I funded. He is helping us avoid the pitfalls that people like us so often run into when they're new to LA and the entertainment industry. He has donated countless hours to help make sure our projects are protected and come to completion. He understands and supports our vision and is a great asset in helping us achieve that vision.

There have been so many people behind the scenes that have helped me get where I am today. I know I'm going to miss some people, and I do not mean any disrespect. Starting with my previous editor, Shannon Leahy, who is a clever and creative writer that helped us with our blogs and editorials. She taught me that when working on a big project like this, the only way to eat an elephant is one piece at a time. Other proofreaders include Leslie McCure, Patricia Evans, MaryTheresa Caprilies, Kari Knapstad, Ondyn Hershel, and Zunaid Vania. For his film and photography in helping us put together the *30 Days of Qigong*, among many other videos, I thank Patrick Monahan. Besides helping us with recording and editing our videos, he has been a loyal friend and supporter for over 16 years. Josh Austin has been crucial in filming, editing, and producing artwork for all our different platforms. Josh is an amazing friend and a wonderful person to work with. Songwriter, composer, and film producer CJ Vanston has been crucial in making sure that our sound and image for The Qi Club is on point. He also has graciously composed music for us and allowed me the opportunity to record Qigong meditations in his studio. He is an amazing friend and I have to pinch myself to realize that I got so lucky to have him walk into my life. I'd like to thank Rizlady and Alex, who filmed, edited, and put together a beautiful sizzle reel for my upcoming TV show. José Ernest Palacios has played a crucial role in book and

CD cover design as well as logo design. He is an amazing and talented artist who has helped us with T-shirt and web design. Jay Menez, host of the show *Hollywood Real* and author of the book *Spark*, has helped me by having me on his show and allowed me to utilize his talents to interview Tae Bo creator Billy Blanks. Besides being a really cool singer and songwriter, Emily Rath helped us with filming videos for our YouTube channel as well as managing our social media platforms. My attorney, Dennis Chui, has helped me out of more than one sticky situation! I thank Brad and Steve, who helped film my first Tai Chi video. Thank you, Eric Iverson, for supporting and maintaining our Qigong Teacher Training website and The Qi Club, as well as building and maintaining the Morning Crane and Shelton Qigong websites. Eric is extremely talented and of all the web developers that we've had, Eric has been by far the easiest to work with. Besides being a really great guy, what I love about Eric is that he always delivers.

Finally, I thank the hundreds of people throughout the years who have played a role directly or indirectly in my success and personal development.

■ ■ ■

FIVE ELEMENT QUESTIONNAIRE

Get Your Five Element Questionnaire by scanning the QR code below or by visiting:

http://chrissheltonseasyguide.com

■ ■ ■

RESOURCES AND RECOMMENDED READING

Chris Shelton's Easy Guide to Emotional Well-Being with Qigong, 3rd ed., by Chris Shelton

Master Tong's Acupuncture: An Ancient Alternative Style in Modern Clinical Practice, by Miriam Lee

Master Tung's Magic Points: A Definitive Clinical Guide, by Susan Johnson and Eric Renaud

The Tao of Nutrition, by Dr. Mao Shing Ni

The Yellow Emperor's Classic of Medicine: A new Translation of the Haungdi Neijing Suwen with Commentary, by Dr. Mao Shing Ni

Live Your Ultimate Life: Ancient Wisdom to Harness Success, Health and Happiness, by Dr. Mao Shing Ni

Face Reading in Chinese Medicine, by Lillian Bridges

The Psoas Book, by Liz Koch

The Book of Changes and the Unchanging Truth, by Hua-Ching Ni

Tao, the Subtle Universal Law, by Hua-Ching Ni

The Web That Has No Weaver, by Ted Kaptchuk

The Foundations of Chinese Medicine, by Giovanni Maciocia

The Practice of Chinese Medicine, by Giovanni Maciocia

Tongue Diagnosis in Chinese Medicine, by Giovanni Maciocia

Fundamentals of Chinese Acupuncture, by Andrew Ellis, Nigel Wiseman, and Ken Boss

Fundamentals of Chinese Medicine, by Nigel Wiseman

The Way to Locate Acupoints, by Yang Jiasan

Super Genes, by Deepak Chopra and Rudolph E. Tanzi

How to Suffer in 10 Easy Steps: Discover, Embrace and Own the Mechanics of Misery, by William Arntz

Healing with Whole Foods, by Paul Pitchford

Clinical Handbook of Internal Medicine, The Treatment of Disease with Traditional Chinese Medicine, Vol. 2: Spleen and Stomach, by Will MacLean

Chinese Dietary Therapy, by Jilin Liu

James Saper, Traditional Chinese Medicine Practitioner, https://www.eastmountain.ca.

■ ■ ■

ACUPUNCTURE POINTS
REFERENCED IN THIS BOOK

The acupuncture points along specific acupuncture meridians have properties that are unique to their nature, location, and function. The acupuncture meridians that include these points are like rivers that feed into the internal organs.

To locate the distance between acupuncture points or from a certain area of the body, the unit of measurement called *cun* is sometimes used. One cun is the width of your thumb at the joint, which is the same width as the middle section of your middle finger. It refers to the thumb of the receiver, not the practitioner. This makes sense because everyone's body size is different and one size doesn't fit all. Thus you can't say something is two inches from a certain point on everyone. Using cun, therefore, allows remedies to be tailored to the individual and their unique physiology.

For example, the acupressure point Kidney 27 is located two cun lateral from the CV channel. Two cun is the same width as the three fingers put together around the first joint. And three cun is the same width as the four fingers put together. One, two, and three. Another faster way to find Kidney 27, which is two cun lateral from the CV channel, is to measure three fingers from the CV channel. So rather than using thumbs all the time, grouping fingers together can sometimes be more efficient.

As you see below, the acupuncture points I use to help with the various types of neck and back issues have many different functions. For example, if you press LV 2 on the Liver channel, between the big toe and second toe, this point also connects to the Heart and can be used for things like heart palpitations and insomnia.

So although your intention is to fix your back problem, utilizing these points will indirectly help rectify other imbalances or illnesses as well.

These acupuncture points and channels not only feed into the internal organs but also help support other organs. They connect the exterior to the interior, the left to the right side of the body, and the upper and lower torso.

Whether you are working on these points yourself or you're a practitioner working with clients, you will find that they support the various strategies listed above to help resolve all types of lower neck and back issues as well as some knee and foot issues.

Abbreviations of the Internal Organs

LV:	Liver	ST:	Stomach
GB:	Gallbladder	LU:	Lungs
HT:	Heart	LI:	Large Intestine
SI:	Small Intestine	KI:	Kidney
PC:	Pericardium	UB:	Urinary Bladder
TB:	Triple Burner	CV:	Conception Vessel
SP:	Spleen	GV:	Governing Vessel

To find the location and function of acupuncture points relevant to back pain, scan the QR code below or visit:

http://chrissheltonseasyguide.com

APPENDIX 4

GLOSSARY

ACUTE   an adjective describing an illness or medical condition characterized by sudden onset of sharp or severe pain, usually of short duration. This can also define someone's emotional state. For example, suddenly losing a loved one can cause intense, acute pain and sorrow.

BI   also referred to as "painful obstruction syndrome," when pathogenic Qi causes blockages in the limbs, trunk, or organs and channels. These patterns normally arise from a combination of wind, cold, and damp type pathogens invading the channels and joints of the body. If there is wind in the body, pain will migrate from various locations to different joints.

BLOOD (XU)   according to Chinese medicine, this has a different meaning than in Western medicine. Blood is a form of Qi. Therefore, when someone has a hard time conceiving of what Qi is, I recommend that they think of their blood. If the blood is deficient or you are anemic, you will lack the vital life force energy, or Qi, needed to carry out even normal activities. Although blood is warm, it is considered yin because it's responsible for providing the nutrients that the body needs. It is also lubricating in nature and helps moisten the eyes and sinews. It helps moisturize the hair on the head, and sweat is an extension of it. Like yin and yang, blood and Qi cannot be separated. It is said that the blood contains Qi and the Qi, in turn, circulates blood throughout the body.

BODY FLUIDS (JIN-YE)   moistening and fluid in nature, derived from food and drink. When separated and transformed by the Spleen, the pure, or clean, fluids move up to the Lungs and down to the Kidneys. The impure are sent down to the Small Intestines and the Urinary Bladder, where they are further separated to help produce substances such as sweat.

CHRONIC   relates to an illness or medical condition characterized by long duration or frequency of recurrence. It continues or occurs again and again, showing little change or extremely slow progression over long periods of time.

CONSCIOUSNESS the awareness of our internal and external existence and our relationship to everything within the multi-universe. It is a part of the intuitive self and when cultivated properly, it allows for the co-manifestation with God, our reality. Some refer to consciousness as awareness, self-awareness, or being awake. It is connected to the mind. When we talk about the mind, we are not talking about the physical location and function of the brain, which is a mere reflection of our reality. It is the intangible part of the self that creates the environment for all-knowingness to develop when one is more present and aware. There are many types of consciousness, and everything in our environment is an extension of that consciousness—the unnameable, the indescribable—which has no distinct shape or form yet takes all shapes and forms, seen and unseen.

CORPOREAL SOUL (PO) connected to the Lungs and associated with the physical aspect of a person's being. The Corporeal Soul's function is to direct the body's physical energies of Zong Qi, Wei Qi, Chen Qi, and Yuan Qi, which are responsible for the proper functioning of the human organism to sustain life. It is said that the Corporeal Soul is the soul that returns to the earth at the time of death. Its energy is dense and heavy.

CURATIVE QIGONG® a holistic medicine practice based upon Five Element Qigong, Tung-style acupuncture, and classical Chinese Medicine. It is an integrated approach to healthcare that works with your emotions, environment, lifestyle habits, and physical functions of your body to understand and reverse the disease and aging process.

DEFICIENT a state in which there is too little of an aspect required for full functioning, i.e., the organ is weak or hypoactive.

DREDGE/DREDGING a technique used in acupuncture, acupressure, and Curative Qigong® wherein you apply pressure to a specific point, massage firmly, and imagine the pain as a dark cloud leaving the channel.

EPIGASTRIC REGION the area of the abdominal region that is superior and central in location, above the umbilicus and between the right and left hypochondria. Some people complain of pain in this area below the sternum on the cartilage of the xiphoid process.

ETHEREAL SOUL (HUN) the soul connected to the Liver that represents the forces within a person that actively manifest as the personality. The Ethereal Soul directs the thinking faculties of both the conscious and unconscious self. It is the proper functioning of the soul that allows us to make plans and execute those plans, and to be creative, expressive, and connected to the energy of life. It is said that the Ethereal Soul is what transcends the body after the death of the physical form.

EXCESS conditions in which there is too much of something, i.e., when an organ is hyperactive.

FIRE the physiology that shows up when yang Qi rises and manifests as signs of heat. This can be from environmental excesses, emotional disturbances, or complete depletion of the body due to overwork, too many orgasms, improper diet, and/or poor lifestyle habits.

FIVE ELEMENTS also referred to as the *wu-hsing*, which is translated as the five phases or passages, or five to go. The designation of the evolutionary phases with the names of the natural elements does not imply a static, insubstantial quality of the phases. The five types of energy transformation have both a dynamic and a static aspect. The dynamic aspect refers to the cyclical transformation of energy that occurs in the natural process of energy movement from which the system of time is derived. The static aspect describes the typical quality of material things and is applied only as classification. The Five Elements are an extension of yin and yang that discern five interacting evolutionary phases (or basic types of energy transformation), which are designated as Earth, Metal, Water, Wood, and Fire. This system provides a complete symbology that illustrates the interrelationships and cyclical transformations of all existence.

FLOATERS a medical condition that affects the eye. There are many possible root causes, including diabetes and Liver dysfunction. They appear as black or gray speckles, strings, or cobwebs that float around when you move your eyes and appear to simply move away if you try to look at them directly.

FLOWERY VISION a medical condition that affects the eye and can be a sign of macular degeneration, stroke, transient ischemic attack (TIA), detached retina, or other conditions. All of these conditions, as well as others causing the symptoms, are connected to Liver dysfunction. Flowery vision manifests in the periphery of the visual field like sunlight reflecting off a lake and ripples of the lake moving around the eye. A person can still see through this episode, especially if they stare straight ahead, as there is a tunnel-like effect while what appear to be waves move in the periphery. A temporary episode can be caused by taking too much vitamin D or the wrong herbal formulas. As a result of the toxins in the Liver, it shows up as symptoms in the eye.

GU QI the first stage of the transformation of food into Qi. Food enters the stomach, is rotted and ripened, and is then transformed into food Qi by the Spleen. This food Qi rises into the chest and combines with the Gathering, Zong, and Original Qi from the Kidneys to be made into blood.

HARMONIZE to bring the body back into homeostasis. To coordinate and bring back into balance one organ with another or with the body as a whole. To balance the yin, yang, Qi, blood, and fluids of the body.

HYPOCHONDRIAC REGION also referred to as the hypochondrium. This describes the region of the abdomen on the left and right sides of the rib cage.

I CHING also referred to as *The Book of Changes and the Unchanging Truth*. Written during a time when wise spiritual teachers began to notice the de-evolution of humankind. The pure minds of the ancient ones had the insight needed to maintain balance in their lives. The answers to the underlying energies in any given situation are derived from the various expressions and interactions of the 64 combinations of yin and yang energies that describe everything in the multi-universe. The I Ching is like an honest friend or teacher who can help safely guide one through the trials of life. It teaches one to look for the most appropriate point in any behavior or event, which is invaluable for an individual's self-discovery, self-alignment, and self-refinement. Through application of the I Ching, one can gain self-mastery and live a wholesome, balanced life. The purpose of the principles of the tool is for one to eventually place the book aside and become their own living I Ching. This would mean they were so in tune with nature (minus the ego) that they could develop an all-knowingness to understand the appropriateness of all situations.

JI QI (WILLPOWER) an energy that is an expression and extension of proper functioning of the Kidneys. If Kidney Qi is strong, we will have the willpower to persevere through challenges and obstacles. Some say that we possess a gene that determines our will to live. The stronger the will, the more intact our Ji Qi.

JING QI (ESSENCE)   the process of refinement. It plays an extremely important role in human physiology. Kidney essence is the most specific type of essence and is derived from both the pre-Heaven and post-Heaven essences. The hereditary energy of a person's constitution is determined by their pre-Heaven essence. However, the Kidney essence interacts with the post-Heaven essence and is therefore replenished by it. This is why it's necessary to take good care of the stomach by consuming healthy and nourishing food and drink.

LATERAL COSTAL REGION   the sides of the rib cage, or the hypochondriac region.

LIFE GATE OF FIRE (MING MEIN)   the motive force between the left and right Kidneys and the root of the Original Qi that flows between them. The Kidneys relate to water and the Gate of Fire, also referred to as the Minister of Fire, providing the motive force necessary to transform water into the steam or mist that circulates up to the chest and around the body.

MAGNET THERAPY   supports regenerative processes, calms the nerves, reduces pain, reduces inflammation, moves Qi, accelerates bone union, moves blood, relieves edema and pain as well as shorten the time needed for recovery. It enables effective pain and edema reduction, and can help even during post-surgery healing phase.

MICROCOSM   a smaller part of a larger system, usually referring to an aspect of the cosmos and multi-universe. The microcosm will always reflect aspects of the macrocosm, and by embracing this understanding we can understand how our thoughts and actions affect all aspects of our existence.

NUTRITIVE QI   also referred to as Ying Qi, which literally translates as Nourishing Qi. It has the responsibility of nourishing the internal organs of the whole body and is closely connected to the blood flow within vessels and channels. This type of Qi is yin in comparison to Defensive Qi.

ORIGINAL QI   the essence of our life but in the form of Qi. It is the origin of the Kidneys and is said to house what is referred to as Original yin and yang, which means that it is the root of yin and yang energies for the entire body. It is the basis of Kidney Qi and aids in the transformation of Gathering Qi to True Qi as well as in the transformation of Food Qi to blood. It determines growth, reproduction, and development. It produces bone and brain marrow and is the foundation for one's underlying constitution, meaning how long we will live and how well we are capable of fighting off disease and stress.

PATHOGEN   any influence opposing the correct functioning of Qi in the body.

POST-HEAVEN QI   the essence that is refined and extracted from food and fluid by the Stomach and Spleen after birth. Once a newborn baby begins to breathe and take in nourishment, its Lungs, Stomach, and Spleen start functioning to produce Qi from food and drink.

PRE-HEAVEN ESSENCE   at the time of conception, the blending of sexual energies belonging to man, woman, the environment, and God, or the Tao. This essence is what predetermines a person's basic constitutional makeup, strength, and vitality. It is what makes the individual unique and is closely linked with the Gate of Fire (Ming Mein) that is situated between the left and right Kidneys. This Gate of Fire is a physiological essence for all the body's processes and for all the internal organs.

QI (CHI)   the life force energy that emanates through all things, seen and unseen. It is formless, elusive, and without tangible qualities yet is the subtle breath of life that permeates the entire universe. Qi gives birth to life and is the generative force of the universe. Everything that exists is a manifestation, or projection, of this energy in a grosser or finer state and at a higher or lower frequency of vibration.

QIGONG   a simple practice of specific, guided, and mindful meditations in combination with gentle movements in order to harness life force energy to bring balance and wholeness to one's physical, mental/emotional, and spiritual being. Qi is life force energy and *Gong* is a skill by which one can learn to harness this energy to improve their quality of life and, at the same time, subtly develop spiritual attainment.

SALLOW COMPLEXION   a yellowish/greenish complexion, often combined with other conditions. For example, a person can have a greasy sallow complexion, a dry sallow complexion, or a withered sallow complexion. This can be due to various dysfunctions of the internal organs, in particular the Spleen and the Liver, and can be a sign of anemia, vitamin deficiency, dehydration, or side effects of smoking.

SHEN (SPIRIT)   directed energy that determines and upholds the specific character of an individual. It is the energy responsible for the organization of the living being. In the West, the closest word to describe this would be *soul*. Shen is what determines, produces, and maintains the configuration of an individual's energy. It is active in every phenomenon and on every evolving level. It is said that the Shen is housed in the Heart and is reflected through the brightness of the eyes.

SUPPLEMENTATION   the process of increasing or strengthening any element of the body that needs it. Supplementation is often associated with Qi when we want to boost energy, particularly of the Spleen and Kidneys. We can also supplement yin and yang, blood, Qi, and fluids. For other organs and areas of the body, we often use terms such as strengthen, invigorate, nourish, and fortify.

TAI CHI (TAIJI)   meaning "grand ultimate" or "grand extreme," it is a series of soft, flowing, and explosive postures that utilize one's structure, proper body alignment, mind intent, and Qi.

TAI CHI (OR TAIJI) SYMBOL   represents two apparent opposites simultaneously existing within one another. They are interdependent, not independent. One cannot exist without the other.

TAIJIQUAN (TAI CHI CHUAN)   a complete martial arts system incorporating Taiji principles rooted in the various manifestations of the two oppositional, yet at the same time reciprocal, energies—yin and yang—which can be observed, explored, and experienced as the substantial and the insubstantial, the soft and the hard, the fast and the slow, the tense and the relaxed, the expanded and the contracted, the open and the closed, etc.

UNMANIFEST   the pure, formless, indescribable, incomprehensible, and absolute being from which creation and manifestation unfolds.

WEI QI (DEFENSIVE QI)   connected to the Lungs and responsible for the body's ability to ward off the intrusion of pathogens. It is a more yang type of Qi in relationship to Nutritive Qi and is the further extension of Zhen Qi of the chest. This Qi of the body circulates through the channels and outside the body. It can be compared to an energetic bubble that surrounds the body and has three layers. The first layer connects to the physical essence of our being and resides one to two inches around the body. The second layer connects to the mental/emotional aspect of our being and is approximately two to three feet around the body. The third layer connects to the spiritual aspect of our being and, on average, will be several feet around the body. This is the part of our intuitive self that can sense or feel someone staring at us. It is said that we're able to feel this because of the other person tapping into that third level of Wei Qi. Besides preventing the intrusion of external pathogens, Wei Qi warms, moistens, and partially nourishes the skin and muscles. It also regulates the opening and closing of the pores of the skin and therefore regulates sweating.

WIND one of the most virulent origins of external causes of disease and the driving force for all disease. It refers not only to external wind but to internal wind as well. Internal wind symptoms can take many forms, from mild to serious, and they have one thing in common—movement. Generally, when we have wind inside our bodies, we have conditions like trigeminal facial neuralgia, eye tremors, epilepsy, and seizures. Restless legs syndrome and shivering can also be signs of wind inside the body and of a disease that keeps changing. It includes chronic pain that migrates from one joint to another, which is called bi syndrome and is often diagnosed as an inflammatory disease like fibromyalgia. Combined with wind, we can have other climatic conditions such as cold and heat. These are external types of wind that can be caused by natural wind, air conditioners, heaters, or even the wind blowing on your face in the car. In Western medicine, this would be considered a cold or flu. The various symptoms that arise as a result tell us if it is a wind cold or a wind heat type of disease.

WUJI also referred to as the Tao, the unmanifest, or God. It is the origin of the creation of Heaven and Earth.

YANG active, moving, and creating, yang represents the immaterial, or intangible, state of Qi—that is, pure energy.

YI QI (INTELLECT) rooted in the Spleen, it is the conscious energy that directs the process of memory. When the Spleen is healthy and in balance, the person's memory will be strong.

YIN also referred to as matter, or the material world. Yin represents the solid and static state of Qi and is subtle and inactive.

UPRIGHT QI (ZHENG QI) a general term to indicate the various types of Qi that protect the body from the invasion of exterior pathogens. In addition to Defensive Qi, Nourishing Qi, and Kidney Qi, it plays a role in protecting the body. Upright Qi is used to contrast the effect of pathogens from the body's ability to defend itself from them.

ZONG QI (GATHERING QI) closely related to the function of the Heart and Lungs. It is this function that is in charge of controlling Qi and breathing while also controlling the blood and blood vessels. It is a more subtle type of Qi than Gu Qi.

PHOTO, IMAGE, AND ILLUSTRATION REFERENCE GUIDE

LUMBAR SPINE

INDEX

WANT TO LEARN MORE?

Check out my other book, *Chris Shelton's Easy Guide to Emotional Well-Being with Qigong*, 3rd ed., and view other extra resources by scanning the QR code below or visiting:

http://chrissheltonseasyguide.com

SHOW SOME LOVE

Love this book? Don't forget to leave a review!

Every review matters, and it matters a lot!

Head over to Amazon, or wherever you purchased this book, to leave an honest review for me.

I thank you endlessly.